I. FOREWORD

Welcome to edition 40 of
Medicines, Ethics and Practice (MEP).

Reflecting the evolution of the Royal Pharmaceutical Society into the professional body for pharmacists on 27 September 2010, and the transfer of regulatory roles to the General Pharmaceutical Council, the MEP continues to evolve.

This professional guide for pharmacists has been designed as an underpinning document to help pharmacists practise confidently and professionally. It embeds professionalism and professional judgement at the heart of the decision-making process.

This continues the MEP's tradition of providing information and guidance on legislation affecting pharmacy practice; supporting day-to-day practice rather than simply highlighting pharmacists' statutory obligations.

The MEP is written by the RPS Professional Support team, a small team of pharmacists and advisors from different pharmacy sectors. The team works in collaboration with specialist colleagues within the professional body and external experts within the profession and produces a range of guidance materials to support members in their day-to-day practice. It also provides online professional support at **www.rpharms.com**, by tel: 0845 257 2570 or 0207 572 2737, or by email: support@rpharms.com.

One copy of MEP is distributed to all RPS Members, Fellows, Associates, Pharmaceutical Scientists and Associate pre-registration trainee members who are due to qualify in 2017. All members, including student members, benefit from free online access and discounted purchase prices. Copies of MEP are available for general purchase at a cost of £55.00 and are available from the Pharmaceutical Press website at **www.pharmpress.com** or from Pharmaceutical Press c/o Macmillan on tel: 01256 302 699.

We welcome comments and feedback; these can be sent to us using the contact details above or by post to RPS Professional Support, Royal Pharmaceutical Society, 66-68 East Smithfield, London E1W 1AW.

DISCLAIMER

This publication is intended as a guide and may not always include all information relating to its subject matter. You should interpret all information and advice in light of your own professional knowledge and all relevant pharmacy and healthcare literature and guidelines. Nothing in this publication constitutes legal advice and cannot be relied upon as such. Whilst care has been taken to ensure the accuracy of content RPSGB excludes to the fullest extent permissible by law any liability whether in contract, tort or otherwise arising from your reliance on any information or advice.

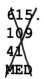

1.1 Changes for this edition

The following significant amendments and additions have been made for edition 40.

New sections

3.3.10.6 Supply of naloxone by individuals employed or engaged in the provision of recognised drug treatment services

3.3.14 Explaining biosimilar medicines

Updated sections

2.3 Professionalism and professional judgement: information on conflicts of interest and declaration of interests

2.4 Clinical check: signposting to new RPS resources on electronic health records

2.5.1 Medicines reconciliation: updated

2.5.2 Helping patients to understand their medicines: updated

2.6 Getting the culture right: signposting to new RPS resources on near miss errors

3.3.6 Military prescriptions: updated

3.3.13 Dispensing valproate for girls and women: updated

3.3.15 Summary of prescriber types and prescribing restrictions: updated to include new information on therapeutic radiographer independent prescribers and dietitian supplementary prescribers

3.3.16 Checking registration of healthcare professionals and additional information on conditions of supply: updated to include new information on sale, supply and administration of medicines by orthoptists

3.4 Wholesale dealing:

■ clarification on Controlled Drugs

■ signposting to information on supply to orthoptists

3.5.8 Reporting adverse events: additional signposting to Yellow Card mobile app

3.5.13 Collection and purchase of medicines by children: updated to include guidance on purchase of medicines by children

3.5.17 Administration of adrenaline in an emergency: updated

3.6 Veterinary medicines: updated information on wholesale dealing (including human medicines for veterinary use under the Cascade)

3.7 Controlled Drugs: updates to reflect new NICE guidance *Controlled drugs: safe use and management* which was published in April 2016

3.7.1 Controlled Drugs – background: updated information on accountable officers

3.7.6 Obtaining Controlled Drugs – requisition requirements for Schedule 1, 2 and 3 Controlled Drugs: updated to reflect changes to legislation

3.7.7 Instalment direction for Schedule 2 and 3 Controlled Drugs: updated to include new Home Office approved wording

3.7.10 Destruction of Controlled Drugs: methods of destruction updated

3.7.11 Record keeping and Controlled Drugs registers: running balances updated

3.7.12 Disposing of spent methadone bottles: updated

CONTENTS

APPENDICES

INDEX

2. CORE CONCEPTS AND SKILLS

This section discusses in detail the core concepts which will equip you with knowledge and skills to help you practise confidently and professionally as a pharmacist.

2.1 Patient or person-centred healthcare

The concept of patient or person-centred healthcare is important to pharmacy and to other health and social care professionals, and has been integrated into healthcare policy throughout Great Britain.

It has been described by different organisations across the globe, all of which have identified common themes such as:

■ Treating patients as equal partners in decisions about their care

■ Putting patients at the centre of all decisions

■ Respect for patient preferences

■ Compassion

■ Dignity

■ Empathy

■ Support for self-care, enablement, autonomy and independence

■ Choice, control and influence

■ Good communication.

Below are some examples of what patient-centred healthcare means in practice:

■ Patients being treated as people

■ Patients being called by the name they prefer and are used to rather than by the name on official documentation (e.g. prefer being called Mike instead of Michael)

■ Being asked to do something and not being told

■ Being able to make informed choices

■ Being able to speak openly about their experiences of taking or not taking medicines, their views about what medicines mean to them, and how medicines impact on their daily life (e.g. when to wake up, when to sleep)

■ Involving patients in decisions about their medicines and self care.

FURTHER READING

The Health Foundation. *Patient-centred care.* (http://personcentredcare.health.org.uk/)

Health in Wales. *Person driven care – Improving Healthcare white paper series No. 7.* (www.1000livesplus.wales.nhs.uk)

NHS Scotland Quality Improvement Hub. *Person centred care.* (www.qihub.scot.nhs.uk/person-centred.aspx)

UK Drug Policy Commission. *Getting serious about stigma: the problem with stigmatising drug users.* (www.ukdpc.org.uk)

BMA, Pharmacy Voice, PSNC. *Joint guidance on prescription direction.* (www.psnc.org.uk)

2.2 Medicines optimisation and pharmaceutical care

Pharmacists have regular contact with patients and are therefore in a key position to spearhead patient centred approaches that enable patients to obtain the best possible outcomes from their medicines as outlined in the medicines optimisation (England), pharmaceutical care (Scotland) and pharmaceutical care and prudent pharmacy (Wales) guidance documents.

The core skills discussed in the MEP can help pharmacists deliver a patient centred approach as outlined in the medicines optimisation, pharmaceutical care and pharmaceutical care and prudent pharmacy guidance.

Medicines optimisation (England)

Medicines optimisation is about ensuring that patients get the best possible outcomes from their medicines. The first step is to ensure that the right patients get the right choice of medicine, at the right time. But the focus needs to be on the individual patient, their beliefs and their experiences. The goal is to help patients to: improve their outcomes; take their medicines correctly and improve adherence; avoid taking unnecessary medicines; reduce wastage of medicines; and improve medicines and patient safety. Ultimately, medicines optimisation can help encourage patients to take ownership of their treatment.

It is a patient-focused approach to getting the best from investment in and use of medicines. It requires a holistic approach, an enhanced level of patient-centred professionalism, and partnership between clinical professionals and a patient.

ELEMENTS OF MEDICINES OPTIMISATION

To empower patients and the public to make the most of medicines healthcare professionals need to understand the concept of medicines optimisation. Diagram 1 outlines the seven elements of medicines optimisation which comprise of the four principles as well as measurement and monitoring, improved patient outcomes, and ensuring a patient-centred approach. These describe medicines optimisation in practice and the outcomes it is intended to impact.

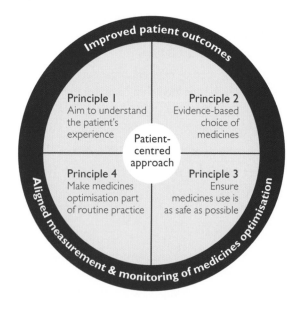

DIAGRAM 1: SUMMARY OF THE FOUR PRINCIPLES OF MEDICINES OPTIMISATION

PRINCIPLE 1: AIM TO UNDERSTAND THE PATIENT'S EXPERIENCE

To ensure the best possible outcomes from medicines, there is an ongoing, open dialogue with the patient and/or their carer about the patient's choice and experience of using medicines to manage their condition; recognising that the patient's experience may change over time even if the medicines do not.

PRINCIPLE 2: EVIDENCE-BASED CHOICE OF MEDICINES

Ensure that the most appropriate choice of clinically and cost-effective medicines (informed by the best available evidence base) are made that can best meet the needs of the patient.

PRINCIPLE 3: ENSURE MEDICINES USE IS AS SAFE AS POSSIBLE

The safe use of medicines is the responsibility of all professionals, healthcare organisations and patients, and should be discussed with patients and/or their carers. Safety covers all aspects of medicines usage, including unwanted effects, interactions, safe processes and systems, and effective communication between professionals.

PRINCIPLE 4: MAKE MEDICINES OPTIMISATION PART OF ROUTINE PRACTICE

Health professionals routinely discuss with each other and with patients and/or their carers how to get the best outcomes from medicines throughout the patient's care.

Further detail on medicines optimisation and the above principles is available on the RPS website in guidance titled *Helping patients make the most of their medicines: Good practice guidance for healthcare professionals in England* **www.rpharms.com/promoting-pharmacy-pdfs/helping-patients-make-the-most-of-their-medicines.pdf**

FURTHER RESOURCES

RPS website. *Medicines optimisation.* **(www.rpharms.com)**

NICE. *Medicines optimisation: the safe and effective use of medicines to enable the best possible outcomes.* 2015. **(www.nice.org.uk)**

Now or Never: Shaping Pharmacy for the Future

In November 2013 the Royal Pharmaceutical Society launched a commission into new models of care through pharmacy. This resulted in the *Now or Never: Shaping Pharmacy for the Future* report. It highlighted that people across England should expect pharmacists to offer more than just medicines and they should play a more integrated role in the healthcare system.

The *Now or Never* report was the first step in a drive to achieve real change for patients and create high quality services at locations that are most convenient for them.

RPS has spent the time since the publication of *Now or Never* looking at how the recommendations of the report can be realised and where pharmacy can have the biggest impact on improving patient care and help the NHS meet the challenge of increased demand from patients for high quality and accessible healthcare in a time of constrained resources.

The following are the key five campaigns which the RPS will pursue as we work to shape pharmacy for the future and improve patient care in England through pharmacy:

- Improving urgent and emergency care through better use of pharmacists
- Pharmacists and GP surgeries
- Pharmacist access to the patient health record
- Pharmacists improving care in care homes
- Pharmacist-led care of people with long term conditions.

Further information (including the report itself and the Nuffield Trust's review of progress one year on *Now more than ever*) can be accessed at **www.rpharms.com/what-we-re-working-on/models-of-care.asp**

Community pharmacy reforms

In response to the Department of Health's letter to PSNC announcing a reduction of at least 6% in funding through the community pharmacy contractual framework, the RPS has developed a community pharmacy reforms hub page: **http://www.rpharms.com/landing-pages/community-pharmacy-reforms.asp**. This has been designed for pharmacists to help them understand the changes to community pharmacy in 2016/17 and beyond, and to answer questions that they may have. It also provides information about the work RPS is doing around this.

Pharmaceutical care (Scotland)

Pharmaceutical care evolved from clinical pharmacy practice in the hospital setting and was defined in 1990 as: 'the responsible provision of drug therapy for the purpose of achieving definite outcomes that improve the patient's quality of life.'[1]

Pharmaceutical care is a person-centred philosophy and practice that aims to optimise the benefits of drug therapy and minimise the risk of drug therapy to patients by providing the framework for pharmacists to apply their knowledge and skills. The pharmacist will assess the pharmaceutical needs of patients and take responsibility for meeting those needs in collaboration with other health and social care professionals.

Key components are, the patient assessment to identify unmet pharmaceutical care needs and issues, the development of a pharmaceutical care plan to document the needs identified, to agree patient outcomes, the actions required or taken and the follow-up required.

In Scotland pharmaceutical care has become the cornerstone of national policy and practice in all settings.[2,3,4,5] Pharmaceutical care is embedded within undergraduate and postgraduate education, the community pharmacy contractual framework and clinical pharmacy services within hospital and primary care, including pharmacist prescribing.[5,6]

In practice, the assessment will identify any pharmaceutical care issues with concordance and sets out to establish within the available information:

■ If the drug therapy and dose is appropriate for the condition in this patient

■ If any additional therapy (drug and non-pharmacological) is required

■ If the drug therapy and dose is safe

■ If the person is suffering from any avoidable side effects

■ If the drug therapy, dose and non-pharmacological therapy are effective and achieving a defined desired outcome.

It is a holistic philosophy and practice that will also identify and address the following needs:

■ Public health, educational, medicines management, non-pharmacological management and changes in clinical need.

REFERENCES AND FURTHER READING

[1] **Hepler CD, Strand LM.** *Opportunities and responsibilities in pharmaceutical care.* American Journal of Hospital Pharmacy, March 1990, Volume 47, pages 533-543.

[2] **Clinical Resource and Audit Group National Health Service in Scotland.** *Clinical Pharmacy in the Hospital Pharmaceutical Service: a Framework for Practice.* 1996.

[3] **Clinical Resource and Audit Group. The Scottish Office.** *Clinical Pharmacy Practice in Primary Care; a framework for the provision of community-based NHS pharmaceutical services.* 1999.

[4] **The Scottish Government.** *The Right Medicine, a strategy for pharmaceutical care in Scotland.* 2002. **(www.gov.scot)**

[5] **The Scottish Government.** *Establishing Effective Therapeutic Partnerships – A generic framework to underpin the Chronic Medication Service element of the Community Pharmacy Contract.* 2010. **(www.gov.scot)**

[6] **Community Pharmacy website.** *Chronic Medication Services.* **(www.communitypharmacy.scot.nhs.uk)**

The Scottish Government. *Prescription for Excellence: A vision and Action Plan for the right Pharmaceutical Care through Integrated Partnerships and Innovations.* 2013. **(www.gov.scot)**

Pharmaceutical care and prudent pharmacy (Wales)

Your Care, Your Medicines: Pharmacy at the heart of patient-centred care presents a vision for pharmacy in Wales.

It is the result of work led by the Welsh Pharmaceutical Committee, the committee responsible for advising the Welsh Government on pharmacy issues. It has been supported by the Royal Pharmaceutical Society with contributions from leaders from all sectors of the profession.

It is an ambition that takes into account the current policy drivers for healthcare in Wales that will contribute to:

- The delivery of prudent healthcare
- A change in culture to encourage greater co-production with patients and collaborative working between health professionals
- A rebalancing of services between health care sectors to deliver an increased primary care based focus

- Creating seamless patient care and closing the gaps between services
- Empowering people to take greater responsibility for their own health and wellbeing.

The model of pharmacy engagement presented in *Your Care, Your Medicines* (Diagram 2) demonstrates patient interactions with the pharmacy team at various points of their health care journey.

The ambition is for patients in Wales to be put at the centre of their care, to benefit from the full integration of the pharmacy team into the NHS and to ensure every intervention involving medicines is supported, communicated and coordinated across the health and social care system.

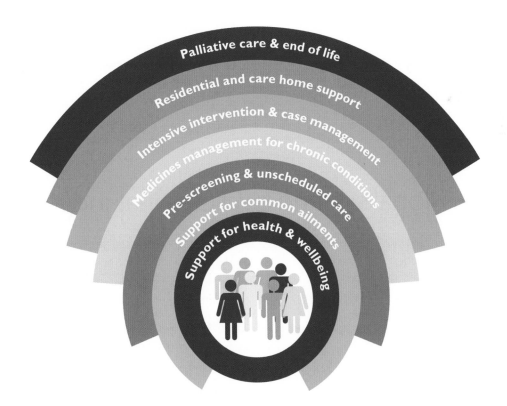

DIAGRAM 2: MODEL OF PHARMACY ENGAGEMENT

The key ambitions in the document are:

AMBITION 1

Patients will routinely access health promotion advice and self-care support from the pharmacy team. This will include healthy lifestyle information, medicines advice and opportunistic interventions at the point of medicines supply. Advances in technology will be exploited to maximise benefits for patients in accessing pharmacy support.

AMBITION 2

The people of Wales will benefit from early detection and treatment of health conditions when engaging with the pharmacy team. Patients will expect the symptoms of minor ailments and non-life threatening emergencies to be treated by the pharmacy team and to be referred to other health services when symptoms require further and more specialised investigation and treatment.

AMBITION 3

Patients with chronic conditions will have regular reviews with a pharmacist who will provide medication advice and coaching in a setting that is most suitable for the patient. A pharmaceutical care plan will be initiated, discussed and jointly managed between the patient and the pharmacist and made available to other health professionals involved in the patient's care.

AMBITION 4

When patients require planned hospital care or any intensive health care they will feel confident that a holistic approach is taken to the management of their conditions and that all decisions on medication changes will be led by expert advice from the pharmacy team.

AMBITION 5

Patients with supported living needs, whether living independently in their own homes or in a care home setting, must benefit from access to the pharmacy team to help manage their medicines effectively and to maintain their health and wellbeing.

AMBITION 6

Patients with palliative care and end of life care needs will be treated with dignity and respect and empowered to shape their clinical pathway with support from the pharmacy team.

FURTHER RESOURCES

RPS website. *Your Care, Your Medicines: Pharmacy at the heart of patient-centred care.* **(www.rpharms.com/what-we-re-working-on/your-care--your-medicines.asp)**

Further information on the prudent agenda can be found at **(www.prudenthealthcare.org.uk)**

2.3 Professionalism and professional judgement

It is important to recognise that pharmacy is not just any occupation; it is a profession and pharmacists are professionals who exercise professionalism and professional judgement on a day-to-day basis.

The concepts of a 'profession', a 'professional' and 'professionalism' are not rigidly defined. However, these are concepts that are important for any pharmacist, including those who work in non-patient facing roles.

A profession can be described as:

- An occupation that is recognised by the public as a profession
- An occupation for which there is a recognised representative professional body
- An occupation that benefits from professional standards and codes of conduct
- An occupation that is regulated to ensure the maintenance of standards and codes of conduct.

A professional can be described as:

- A member of a profession
- A member of a professional body.

An individual who:

- Behaves and acts professionally
- Exercises professionalism and professional judgement, and
- Has professional values, attitudes and behaviours.

Professionalism

Pharmacy professionalism can be defined as a set of values, behaviours and relationships that underpin the trust the public has in pharmacists. Examples of these are:

- Altruism
- Appropriate accountability
- Compassion
- Duty
- Excellence and continuous improvement
- Honour and integrity
- Professional judgement
- Respect for other patients, colleagues and other healthcare professionals
- Working in partnership with patients, doctors and the wider healthcare team in the patient's/public's best interest.

Many of these values, attitudes and behaviours are also reflected in the mandatory GPhC Standards for Conduct, Ethics and Performance (see Appendix 1). Pharmacists who are working in industry should also adhere to the ABPI Code of Practice for the Pharmaceutical Industry (www.abpi.org.uk).

Pharmacists who are working in hospitals, or who are providing services to care homes and other regulated healthcare settings should also be aware of their requirements to comply with the Care Quality Commission (CQC) standards in England (http://www.cqc.org.uk/content/regulations-service-providers-and-managers), Healthcare Improvement Scotland (HIS) standards in Scotland (http://healthcareimprovementscotland.org/), and Healthcare Inspectorate Wales (HIW) standards in Wales (http://www.hiw.org.uk/regulate-healthcare-1).

Conflicts of interest and declaration of interests

The GPhC Standards for Conduct Ethics and Performance require pharmacists to:

Avoid conflicts of interest and declare any personal or professional interests you have. Do not ask for or accept gifts, rewards or hospitality that may affect, or be seen to affect, your professional judgement.

All RPS members should avoid conflicts of interest and if a situation arises where others could perceive that they have competing interests, and/or that their judgement could be influenced or impaired, the individual should ensure that they declare any interests that they have to those who may be affected. The aim of declaring interests is to support transparency. Personal and non-personal matters should be declared which, in the perception of others, might be seen to give material or other advantage (financial or non-financial) to the individual concerned or her/his close family members, either directly or indirectly (for example to a business or another organisation). Individuals should also declare relevant interests where there may be a perception of conflicting loyalty (for example, where the individual is employed by, or has an affiliation with an organisation).

Declaration of an interest does not necessarily prevent an individual from carrying out a role, but it ensures that there can be no perception that they may be seeking improperly to influence decisions.

Professional judgement

Professional judgement can be described as the use of accumulated knowledge and experience, as well as critical reasoning, to make an informed professional decision – often to solve or ameliorate a problem presented by, or in relation to, a patient; or policies and procedures affecting patients. It takes into account the law, ethical considerations, relevant standards and all other relevant factors related to the surrounding circumstances. Furthermore, it will resonate with the core values, attitudes and behavioural indicators of professionalism.

How do I exercise professional judgement?

Many pharmacists exercise their professional judgement instinctively but it may be helpful to break the process down into smaller steps:

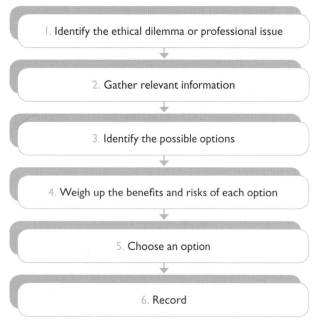

1. Identify the ethical dilemma or professional issue

2. Gather relevant information

3. Identify the possible options

4. Weigh up the benefits and risks of each option

5. Choose an option

6. Record

DiAGRAM 3: EXERCISING PROFESSIONAL JUDGEMENT

1. Identify the ethical dilemma or professional issue you are faced with, e.g. deciding whether to supply a medicine or not.

2. Gather all the relevant information and research the problem – i.e. obtain the following:

   ■ Facts

   ■ Knowledge

   ■ Laws

   ■ Standards

   ■ Good practice guidance

   ■ Advice from support services, head office, line managers or colleagues.

3. Identify all the possible options.

4. Weigh up all the benefits and risks, advantages and disadvantages of each of the possible options you have identified.

5. Choose an option. It is important you can justify the decision you have made because often when faced with an ethical dilemma or professional issue pharmacists are weighing up conflicting obligations which could be genuine patient interest, legal obligations, professional standards, public interest, contractual Terms of Service and company policies.

6. It is important to make a record of the decision-making process and your reasons leading to a particular course of action where appropriate. This may be a record in the patient's medication record (PMR), medical record, the back of the prescription register or an intervention record book. This is important as evidence of the thought processes leading to a decision.

It is entirely possible for two different pharmacists, faced with the same facts and circumstances, to choose two different courses of action. This is the nature of a finely balanced ethical dilemma. Both options could be justifiable and legitimate choices for a significant proportion of pharmacists if faced with the same dilemma.

It is important to point out that professional judgement is not a blanket defence or a blanket reason to take the most convenient choice. It must be exercised properly, logically and for valid reasons. If there are mechanisms to achieve the required goal it is foolish to choose an illegal alternative. For example, lending medication would be very difficult to justify if an emergency supply could have been used.

The process of making a professional judgement is underpinned by knowledge. The following chapters of the MEP provide information on the core knowledge required by pharmacists in their day to day practice.

REFERENCES AND FURTHER READING

American Board of Internal Medicine. *Project Professionalism* (7th printing). Philadelphia: the board; 2001.

Appelbe GE, Wingfield J, editors. *Dale and Applebe's Pharmacy and Medicines Law.* 10th edition. London: Pharmaceutical Press; 2013.

Elvey R, Lewis P, Schafheutle E, Willis S, Harrison S, Hassel K. *Patient-centred professionalism among newly registered pharmacists.* 2011. (http://www.pharmacyresearchuk.org) select the Our research and Download a report tabs.

Pharmacy Law and Ethics Association (PLEA). An independent group and a partner of the Royal Pharmaceutical Society of persons interested in pharmacy, law and ethics. The PLEA virtual network is available to PLEA subscribers on the RPS website **(www.rpharms.com)**

Royal College of Physicians working party. *Doctors in society: Medical professionalism in a changing world.* London: the college; 2005.

Schafheutle E, Hassell K, Ashcroft D, et al. *Professionalism in pharmacy education.* 2010. **(http://www.pharmacyresearchuk.org)** select the Our research and Download a report tabs.

Wingfield J, Badcott D. *Pharmacy Ethics and Decision Making.* London: Pharmaceutical Press; 2007.

Association of the British Pharmaceutical Industry. *Disclosure of payments to individual healthcare professionals.* 2015. **(www.abpi.org.uk)**

General Medical Council. *Financial and commercial arrangements and conflicts of interest.* 2013. **(www.gmc-uk.org)**

NHS England. At time of writing NHS England was in the process of strengthening their statutory guidance on managing conflicts of interests for clinical commissioning groups. More information on this project is available on their website. **(https://www.england.nhs.uk/commissioning/pc-co-comms/coi/)**

CORE CONCEPTS AND SKILLS

2.3.1 SOCIAL MEDIA

Pharmacists and aspiring pharmacists who use social media* and social networking* should do so responsibly and with the same high standards which they would apply in real-world interactions.

It is important to maintain proper professional boundaries in relationships and interactions with patients and at all times to respect the confidentiality of others, including patients and colleagues.

Be aware of the potential audience of your online activity, and that this may be publicly accessible, circulated and shared beyond your control. This activity could impact upon your professional image and the reputation of the profession as a whole. Pharmacists should also ensure that they understand and follow company or NHS Trust policies on social media.

The General Pharmaceutical Council (GPhC) *Standards of Conduct, Ethics and Performance* (see Appendix 1) include Standards which require pharmacists to:

Treat people politely and considerately.

AND

Maintain proper professional boundaries in your relationships with patients and others that you come into contact with during the course of your professional practice and take special care when dealing with vulnerable people.

The GPhC have also published *Guidance on Maintaining Clear Sexual Boundaries* and on *Patient Confidentiality* – the latter explicitly states that pharmacists *must not disclose information on any websites, internet chat forums or social media that could identify a patient.*

GPhC Standards also require pharmacists to:

Avoid conflicts of interest and declare any personal or professional interests you have.

AND

Be accurate and impartial when you teach and when you provide or publish information. Do not mislead or make claims that you have no evidence for or cannot justify.

These Standards and Guidance apply on social media*, as well as in the real world and also apply to those who blog anonymously.

*Social media includes blogging, web forums including professional web forums, Twitter, Facebook, online and virtual networks (this list is not exhaustive).

REFERENCES AND FURTHER READING

The RPS has published a multimedia package of social media guidance for pharmacists, it can be viewed on our website at (www.rpharms. com/unsecure-support-resources/social-media-guidance.asp). The information within this guidance is to help pharmacists use social media for the benefit of their practice, the profession, patients and the public.

GPhC. *Standards of Conduct Ethics and Practice.* (www.pharmacyregulation.org) (see Appendix 1)

GPhC. *Guidance on Maintaining Clear Sexual Boundaries.* (www.pharmacyregulation.org) (see Appendix 7)

GPhC. *Guidance on Patient Confidentiality.* (www.pharmacyregulation.org) (see Appendix 4)

British Medical Association. *Social Media Use: Practical and Ethical Guidance for doctors and Medical Students.* (www.bma.org.uk)

Royal College of General Practitioners. *Social Media Highway Code.* (www.rcgp.org.uk)

2.4 Clinical check

One of the key skills of a pharmacist when supplying medicines to patients is to perform a fundamental clinical assessment or clinical check of the medicine to be supplied. Clinical checks involve identifying potential pharmacotherapeutic problems by collating and evaluating all relevant information, including patient characteristics, disease states, medication regimen and, where possible, laboratory results.

Importantly, it is not a mere dose and interaction check, or a simple tick box exercise but rather a complex skill which will often require interaction with patients and healthcare professionals. A clinical check is underpinned by knowledge of human pathophysiology as well as medicines (pharmacokinetics, pharmacology, pharmaceutics, pharmacognosy) coupled with clinical experience and the rational application of professional judgement. It is a key part of clinical pharmacy contributing to patient safety and public health.

Recent evidence-based studies including EQUIP by Dornan et al. which looked at causes of prescribing errors and the PINCER trial by Avery et al. which looked at pharmacist-led technology enabled interventions, highlight the benefit of the clinical input by pharmacists. The PRACtICe study commissioned by the GMC found that pharmacists have a great role in preventing the occurrence of errors through reviewing patients' medicines and identifying and informing the GP of errors at the point of dispensing (www.gmc-uk.org).

By using a structured, logical approach to a clinical check, pharmacists can balance the risks and benefits of a prescribed medicine regimen and, in doing so, improve the medicine's safety and effectiveness.

ELECTRONIC HEALTH RECORDS

Pharmacy access to patient electronic health records provides a way to access patient information that is required to provide pharmacy services.

Various electronic health records are used by pharmacists in daily practice, from the patient medication records that are in routine use in pharmacies, to the national summary records that are being rolled out and piloted in some areas. Further information on the use of Summary Care Records in England, Emergency Care Summary in Scotland and Welsh GP Record are available on the RPS Electronic Health Records section of the RPS website (http://www.rpharms. com/unsecure-support-resources/electronic-health-records.asp). This also includes a decision tool *Using electronic health records (EHR) professionally.*

The sources for obtaining information, and the level of detail available, will vary depending on the pharmacy setting. It may not always be practicable to obtain all the information needed and, sometimes, decisions will need to be made on limited information. Pharmacists should consider the level of risk when deciding if further information is required from one or more additional sources.

In primary care, you may be able to obtain information from:

- The prescription
- The patient, patient's representative or carer

- The patient's GP or other healthcare professionals involved in the patient's care
- The patient's medication record
- Other patient medical records where available (e.g. in Scotland – access to the Emergency Care Summary; access to the Summary Care Record where available; in a prison – access to medical records).

In secondary care, additional sources of information available would include other healthcare professionals involved in the patient's care (e.g. dieticians, microbiologists and physiotherapists), medical and nursing care notes, additional ward charts and laboratory results.

The areas that pharmacists need to consider when undertaking a clinical check include:

- Patient characteristics
- Medication regimen
- How treatment will be administered and monitored.

Patient characteristics

Factors relating to patient characteristics that should be considered during a clinical check include:

- **PATIENT TYPE** – establish whether the patient falls into a group where treatment is contraindicated or cautioned. Specific groups of patients to be aware of include:
  - Children
  - Women who are pregnant or breastfeeding
  - The elderly
  - Certain ethnic groups – a patient's ethnic origin can affect the choice of medicine or dose (e.g. the initial and maximum dose of rosuvastatin is lower for patients of Asian origin).

(For some medicines, the gender of the patient should be considered. For example, finasteride is contraindicated for women.)

- **CO-MORBIDITIES** – patient co-morbidities, such as renal or hepatic impairment or heart failure,

can exclude the use of a particular treatment or necessitate dose adjustments

- **PATIENT INTOLERANCES AND PREFERENCES** – other patient factors that can affect the choice of treatment include known medication adverse events (e.g. allergies), dietary intolerances (e.g. to lactose-containing products), patient preferences (e.g. vegan patients may refuse products of porcine origin), religious beliefs, and patients' knowledge and understanding of medicines and why they are being taken (patient beliefs about medicines).

Medication regimen factors

Aspects of the prescribed medication regimen that should be considered during a clinical check include:

- **INDICATION** – ascertain the indication for treatment to check whether the medicine prescribed is appropriate for the indication and compatible with recommended guidelines
- **CHANGES IN REGULAR TREATMENT** – where there are changes in regular therapy (e.g. strength or dose), pharmacists should confirm that these are intentional
- **DOSE, FREQUENCY AND STRENGTH** – pharmacists should check that the dose, frequency and strength of the prescribed medicine are appropriate

– having considered the patient's age, renal and hepatic function, weight (and surface area where appropriate), co-morbidities, concomitant drug treatments and lifestyle pattern

■ **THE DOSING OF THE FORMULATION** – check that, for the formulation prescribed, the dose and frequency are appropriate

■ **DRUG COMPATIBILITY** – regular and new therapies should be evaluated for any clinically significant interactions, duplications and antagonistic activity

■ **MONITORING REQUIREMENTS** – for medicines that require monitoring, pharmacists should check for the latest test results and ascertain whether any dose adjustments are required.

Administration and monitoring

Aspects relating to the administration and monitoring of a medicine that should be considered during a clinical check include:

■ **THE ROUTE OF ADMINISTRATION** – check whether the prescribed route of administration is suitable for the patient and whether a preparation is available for that route. Also, check for compatibility issues that may arise from administering via that route (e.g. due to co-administration of food or other medicines). For example, phenytoin can interact with enteral feeds so administration via an enteral feeding tube would need to be managed accordingly.

■ **THE NEED FOR ADMINISTRATION AIDS** – check whether any adherence aids required by the patient are available. For example, spacer devices, eye drop devices, Braille or large type or pictogram labels, additional information sheets or verbal information.

Record keeping

Record keeping is important for continuity of care, evidence of the benefit of pharmacy input and improving patient care. Pharmacists should make a record of significant clinical checks, and interventions made. This should include details of discussions and agreed decisions with other healthcare professionals. Depending upon the circumstances it may be appropriate to make this record in the patient's medication record (PMR), an interventions record book, handover record book or prescription register.

REFERENCES AND FURTHER READING

British National Formulary
(**www.medicinescomplete.com** or **www.evidence.nhs.uk**)

British National Formulary for Children
(**www.medicinescomplete.com** or **www.evidence.nhs.uk**)

Clinical Pharmacist
(**www.pharmaceutical-journal.com/publications/clinical-pharmacist**)

Stephens M. *Hospital Pharmacy* (2nd edition). London: Pharmaceutical Press; 2011.

Gray AH, Wright J, Bruce L, Oakley J. *Clinical Pharmacy Pocket Companion* (2nd edition). London: Pharmaceutical Press; 2015.

RPS. *Clinical check quick reference guide.* 2011. (**www.rpharms.com/resources-AtoZ**)

Dornan T. et al. *An in depth investigation into causes of prescribing errors by foundation trainees in relation to their medical education. EQUIP Study.* General Medical Council; 2009.

Avery AJ. et al. *Pharmacist-led information technology-enabled intervention for reducing medication errors: Multi-centre cluster randomised controlled trial and cost-effectiveness analysis (PINCER Trial).* The Lancet. 2012.

Avery, AJ. et al. *Investigating the prevalence and causes of prescribing errors in general practice: The PRACtICe Study.* General Medical Council; 2012.

GPhC. *Guidance on consent.* (**www.pharmacyregulation.org**) (see Appendix 5)

RPS. *Quick reference guides under Pharmacy practice and Clinical aspects of pharmacy.* (**www.rpharms.com**)

2.5 The pharmacist consultation in practice

A pharmacist consultation is any discussion between a pharmacist and a patient and the consultation is an essential part of providing patient-centred care in practice. Patients should be encouraged to engage in the consultation to ensure that it is a two-way discussion where they can share their views and be involved in decision-making around their treatment.

The Consultation Skills Assessment (also known as the Medication Related Consultation Framework) is one of the Foundation Pharmacy Framework tools and can be used to assess and demonstrate your consultation behaviours and skills. Further information can be found in the Foundation programme area on the RPS website **http://www.rpharms.com/development/foundation-practice.asp.**

2.5.1 MEDICINES RECONCILIATION

Medicines reconciliation is the process of identifying an accurate list of a patient's current medicines (including over-the-counter and complementary medicines) and carrying out a comparison of these with the current list in use, recognising any discrepancies, and documenting any changes. It also takes into account the current health of the patient and any active or long-standing issues. The result is a complete list of medicines that is then accurately communicated. The pharmacist who is carrying out medicines reconciliation should ensure that any discrepancies are resolved by highlighting these to and working with relevant members of the multidisciplinary team. The pharmacist should also keep the patient informed.

Medicines reconciliation should take place whenever patients are transferred from one care setting to another, when they are admitted to hospital, transferred between wards and on discharge. The way that the process is carried out will vary between care settings. Further information on medicines reconciliation in different settings can be found in NICE Guideline *Medicines optimisation: the safe and effective use of medicines to enable the best possible outcomes:* **https://www.nice.org.uk/guidance/ng5**

Accurate medicines reconciliation prevents medication errors and provides a foundation for assessing the appropriateness of a patient's current medicines and directing future treatment choices to ensure that the patient receive the best care. The process also allows other pharmaceutical issues such as poor adherence or non-adherence to be identified.

Sources of information

Sources of information that may be used when carrying out medicines reconciliation include:

1. Patient or patient's representative
2. Patient's medicines
3. Repeat prescriptions
4. GP referral letters
5. The patient's GP surgery
6. Hospital discharge summaries or outpatient appointment notes
7. Community pharmacy patient medication records
8. Care home records
9. Drug treatment centre records
10. Other healthcare professionals and specialist clinics
11. Patient medical records where available (e.g. in prisons or the Emergency Care Summary (Scotland), Summary Care Record (England), or Welsh GP Record (see also section 2.4).

GENERAL TIPS FOR OBTAINING A MEDICATION HISTORY FROM A PATIENT

- Explain to the patient why the history is being taken

- Use a balance of open-ended questions (e.g. what, how, why, when) with closed questions (i.e. those requiring yes/no answers)

- Avoid jargon – keep it simple

- Clarify vague responses with further questioning or by using other sources of information

- Keep the patient at ease.

Key points

ARE THE SOURCES YOU USE UP-TO-DATE? Aim to use the most complete, reliable and up-to-date source(s) of information.

CROSS-CHECK ADHERENCE Medication histories should be cross-checked against different sources and confirmed with the patient or patient's representative. The medicines they are actually taking, and how they are taking them, may differ from written documentation (e.g. the prescribing record held by the patient's GP).

NON-DAILY MEDICINES Remember to ask patients whether they take any medicines 'when required' (e.g. reliever inhalers), or on certain days of the week. Also remember to ask about the sorts of formulations that might be forgotten (e.g. nasal sprays, eye or ear drops, ointments, depot injections, patches, etc). Patients may also need prompting to remember medicines such as oral contraceptives and hormone replacement therapy.

HISTORICAL MEDICINES The medication history should not be restricted to current therapies but should include any recently stopped or changed medicines.

SELF-SELECTED MEDICINES Include any medicinal product that the patient is taking – whether prescribed or not – and do not restrict the medication history to medicines obtained on prescription. Over-the-counter (OTC) medicines, herbal products, vitamins, dietary supplements, recreational drugs (e.g. alcohol and tobacco) and remedies purchased over the internet should also be included.

What information should I obtain when taking a medication history?

For each medicine, the following should be determined:

- Generic name of the drug

- Brand name of the drug, where appropriate (for example, where bioavailability variations between brands can have clinical consequences, such as lithium therapy)

- Dose – both the prescribed dose and the actual dose the patient is taking (NB: This may best be described to the patient as a quantity of tablets rather than as milligrams of active ingredient)

- Strength of the medicine taken

- Formulation used (e.g. phenytoin – 100mg as a liquid does not deliver the same dose as a 100mg tablet)

- Route of administration (this could be an unlicensed route – e.g. ciprofloxacin eye drops for the ear)

- Frequency of administration – this should include the time of administration for certain medicines (e.g. levodopa)

- Length of therapy, if appropriate (e.g. for antibiotics)

- Administration device and brand for injectables (e.g. insulin)

- Day or date of administration for medicines taken on specific days of the week or month.

FURTHER READING

Stephens M. *Hospital Pharmacy* (2nd edition). London: Pharmaceutical Press; 2011.

RPS. *Medication history – quick reference guide.* 2011. (**www.rpharms.com/resources-AtoZ**)

NICE. *Medicines optimisation: the safe and effective use of medicines to enable the best possible outcomes.* 2015. (**www.nice.org.uk**)

East and South East England Specialist Pharmacy Services. *Medicines reconciliation: Best practice resource and toolkit.* June 2015. (**www.medicinesresources.nhs.uk/en/Communities/NHS/SPS-E-and-SE-England/Meds-use-and-safety/Service-deliv-and-devel/**)

Healthcare Improvement Scotland. *Medicines reconciliation care bundle.* June 2015. (**www.scottishpatientsafetyprogramme.scot.nhs.uk/programmes/primary-care/safer-medicines**)

2.5.2 HELPING PATIENTS TO UNDERSTAND THEIR MEDICINES

An important key role of pharmacists is ensuring that patients understand their medicines, the role that they play in maintaining their wellbeing and to empower patients to use these safely and effectively to get the most from their treatment. Providing information for patients on their medicines involves being able to build a rapport with the patient, having good communication skills, empathy, being able to put the patient at ease and being able to confer an understanding and belief that the health of the patient is important to the pharmacist. Involving and engaging the patient in this process is essential in ensuring that the pharmacist-patient relationship is concordant.

Opportunities for helping patients understand their medicines

Consultations should not be limited to when a supply of newly prescribed medicines is made, and almost any interaction with the patient can be used as an opportunity to help them understand their medicines. A simple question asking, "How are you getting on with your medicines" can often be a successful engaging starting point. Illustrative examples of opportunities include:

- Point of sale for over-the-counter medicines
- Any medication reviews
- Diagnostic testing and screening
- Patient group directions
- Minor ailment schemes
- Whilst taking medication history
- During a hospital stay
- Point of discharge
- Outpatient clinics
- When a change has been made to a current medicine
- Point of a supply of a regular prescription.

Advice for successful patient consultations

- Try to understand the level of existing knowledge, understanding and concerns the patient has regarding their medicines. Consider any misunderstandings which could be a barrier to adherence. Explore what the patient has already been told about their medicines, whether there are any concerns and what the patient's expectations are
- Ensure you are familiar with the medicines you will be providing counselling on and any additional information that is relevant to those medicines. If in doubt, take time to review and re-familiarise yourself with the medicine. For example – look out for interactions with other medicines, food, or supplements, or medicines with common or significant side effects, complex administration regimens, special storage requirements, or narrow therapeutic index. Check standard

references (e.g. BNF or national guidelines for additional patient and carer advice)

- Aim for a structured approach and tailor the language and level of detail used to the patient. The format that is appropriate will depend upon both patient characteristics and the medicines that are taken. As an illustration, the patient may be knowledgeable about their medicines and condition, for example as a result of caring for a family member with the same condition

- Where appropriate use different methods of communication to support your discussions such as pictograms and medication cards

- Respect patient privacy and ensure that confidentiality is protected

- Ensure that the process is two-way and interactive, not simply a list of facts about medicines. There should be opportunities for questions and discussion.

As a minimum, you should consider discussing the following points:

- What is the medicine and why has it been prescribed? How does it impact upon the medical condition and how does it alleviate the symptoms? e.g. This is a blood pressure medicine which should lower your blood pressure to normal levels which will help prevent further complications

- How and when to take the medicine

- How much to take and what to expect, e.g. antibiotics need to be taken regularly and the course completed even after symptoms subside

- What to do if the patient misses a dose

- What are the likely side effects and how to manage them

- If applicable, any lifestyle or dietary changes that need to be made or that can affect the treatment

- Additional information relating to storage requirements, expiry dates, disposal and monitoring requirements can also be included where appropriate

- Check patient understanding by asking them to describe back to you the key information you have provided.

REFERENCES AND FURTHER RESOURCES

CPPE. *Consultation skills for pharmacy practice: Taking a patient-centered approach.* 2014. **(www.cppe.ac.uk)**

WCPPE. *Consultation skills for pharmacy practice: Taking a patient-centered approach.* 2015. **(www.wcppe.org.uk)**

NHS Education for Scotland. *Patient centred consultation skills training* (one day training course). **(www.nes.scot.nhs.uk/education-and-training/by-discipline/pharmacy.aspx)**

CPPE. *Confidence in consultation skills* (a workshop for pharmacists). **(www.cppe.ac.uk)**

CPPE and NHS Health Education England. *Consultation skills for pharmacy practice: practice standards for England.* 2014. **(www.consultationskillsforpharmacy.com)** (Endorsed by the RPS)

NICE guidance. *Medicines adherence: Involving patients in decisions about prescribed medicines and supporting adherence.* **(www.nice.org.uk)**

RPS. *Medication review – quick reference guide.* **(www.rpharms.com/resources-AtoZ)**

RPS. *Medicines adherence – quick reference guide.* **(www.rpharms.com/resources-AtoZ)**

Hugman, Bruce. *Healthcare communication* (1st edition). London: Pharmaceutical Press; 2009.

RPS. *Counselling patients – quick reference guide.* **(www.rpharms.com/resources-AtoZ)**

GP-training.net. *Communication skills resources and concise information regarding the Cambridge-Calgary model.* **(www.gp-training.net)**

2.6 Getting the culture right

"In the end, culture will trump rules, standards and control strategies every single time." Professor Donald Berwick. A promise to learn – a commitment to act (2013)

We know that it is important for the profession to get the culture right. There have been infamous examples across industries and organisations of the problems caused by the wrong culture, including within the banking industry, the media and within healthcare. The wrong type of culture contributed to the unacceptable failings at Mid-Staffordshire NHS Foundation Trust hospital between 2005 and 2008, those at Orchid View care home and also the abuse at Winterbourne View private hospital.

The types of culture which collectively help us to achieve patient-centred, safe and effective care together with professional empowerment are interlinked and include a culture that is based upon the principles and values of fairness, quality, safety, transparency, learning and reporting.

Underpinning getting the culture right is a '*just culture*'. This is a culture based upon fairness and is achieved when attitudes, behaviours and practices are fair.

2.6.1 A JUST CULTURE

PROBLEMS WITH A PUNITIVE CULTURE

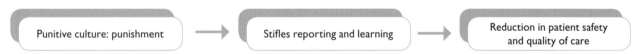

A *punitive culture* is based upon assigning blame and punishment. It contributes to creating a culture of fear. People and organisations see what happens to others and if what they see is perceived to be draconian or unjust, this leads to fear, stifling reporting and stifling the raising of concerns. We lose the opportunity to learn, and patient safety is affected. A single instance of perceived punitive action can have a wide effect on how large groups of people choose to act.

WHY A NO-BLAME CULTURE IS INADEQUATE

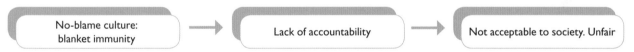

A *no-blame* culture may not be better than a *punitive culture*. It can breed complacency or nonchalance which can also impact upon patient safety. At its worst it can appear unacceptable to society overall due to the immunity from accountability which can also be abused. For example, there is a perception that at times diplomatic immunity can be unfair and abused.

THE 'RIGHT CULTURE' OR A JUST CULTURE

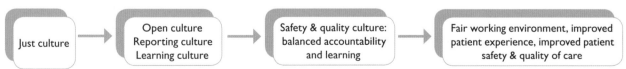

Instead, the 'right culture' is needed which is a culture based upon the principles of fairness, quality, transparency, reporting, learning and safety.

A *just culture* promotes an open culture (transparency and discussion), a reporting culture (raising concerns), and a learning culture (learning from mistakes). These cultures support each other to create a safety culture – balancing accountability and learning and leading to improved patient safety. It also creates a just and open working environment which is rewarding to work in, fosters professional empowerment, and enhances the quality of service to patients and the patient experience.

Why is it needed?

When applied to the provision of healthcare and pharmacy services, a *just culture* means removing fears, increasing sharing and reporting of concerns, being able to learn from mistakes or incidents, being able to share lessons learnt (throughout the profession where appropriate) and using this shared learning to reduce the likelihood of similar mistakes and incidents happening again. This is a vital component contributing to better patient safety.

When a mistake or incident occurs, we all want assurances that actions are being taken so that it will never happen again and that there will be fair accountability. It is not possible to stop errors occurring, however, a *just culture* will contribute to a system that improves continuously which should in time result in fewer errors.

HOW DO WE COLLECTIVELY ACHIEVE A JUST CULTURE?

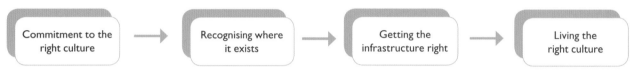

Commitment to the right culture → Recognising where it exists → Getting the infrastructure right → Living the right culture

The journey to achieving the right culture requires the embedding of *just culture* principles into attitudes, behaviours and practices, and the design of legislation, regulation, standards, policies and systems.

It requires commitment by all stakeholders to apply and 'live' the culture routinely, through all activities and all interfaces and for this to be habitual. It is a continuous and evolving movement and may take years to achieve, but one to which the Royal Pharmaceutical Society and others are committed. Policies and procedures for a just and safe culture are simply words on paper if they are not 'lived' in actions and interactions. We all have responsibilities for living the culture and embedding the habit. Individuals and

organisations can do this through strong leadership and educating people about a just and safe culture appreciating when it is in action through reflection, through benchmarking and through commitment of time.

In October 2012, on behalf of the profession, the Royal Pharmaceutical Society was instrumental in designing and creating *The Speaking Up Charter* together with NHS Employers and other stakeholders. This charter incorporates *just culture* ideals and has been supported by major healthcare organisations. (**http://www.nhsemployers. org/your-workforce/retain-and-improve/raising-concerns- at-work-and-whistleblowing/information-for-employers/ speaking-up-charter**)

A *just culture* and patient safety incidents

Patient safety can be improved by the reporting of concerns and learning from these reports. The reporting of concerns will only take place if individuals feel they will not be victimised and that it is 'safe' to report these concerns. To provide assurance and confidence, everybody needs to know where they stand.

The airline industry has been embedding *just culture* principles into its practices for decades to improve safety.

Adapting from what the airline industry has learnt, together with consideration of similar workstreams within the NHS, we believe in the following *just culture* principles for patient safety incidents:

1. Patient safety is paramount.

2. Deliberate harm and unacceptable risk impacting on patient safety must not be tolerated.

3. Patient safety is maintained by healthcare professionals being candid and raising concerns and learning from incidents to improve systems, standards, policies, legislation and people.

4. To ensure that concerns will be raised and learning from incidents occurs, individual accountability must always be fair and proportionate, and viewed in the context of root cause, system deficiencies, mitigating circumstances and the entirety of contributing factors (i.e. the whole picture).

The NHS has developed an incident decision tree (see Diagram 4) based upon the work of Professor James Reason, an expert on patient safety. This decision-making tool embodies *just culture* principles and uses a series of tests to decide on the appropriate course of action following an incident.

NATIONAL REPORTING AND LEARNING SYSTEM (NRLS)

From June 2012 the key functions for patient safety developed by the National Patient Safety Agency (NPSA) were transferred to the NHS Commissioning Board Special Health Authority. The NPSA website continues to offer key information, guidance, tools and alerts. Healthcare organisations in England and Wales should report patient safety incidents to the NRLS **(http://www. nrls.npsa.nhs.uk/report-a-patient-safety-incident/)**. The NRLS does not seek to collect identifiable information relating to staff and patients involved in an incident and so reporting is anonymous for the reporter, staff and patients.

In Scotland each NHS Board operates its own reporting system.

NEAR MISS ERRORS

Regular review of near miss errors and action taken can prevent similar mistakes from happening in the future. The RPS has produced tools and guidance to help support clinical governance in pharmacy, and to promote an open culture of recording of near miss errors so that all pharmacy staff can reflect and learn from them. The Near Miss Error Log and Near Miss Error Improvement Tool, along with supporting guidance are available on the RPS website **(http://www.rpharms.com/unsecure-support-resources/near-miss-errors.asp)**.

Decker S. *Just Culture: Balancing Safety and Accountability.* (2nd edition). Ashgate; 2012.

Meadows S, Baker K, Butler J. *The incident decision tree: guidelines for action following patient safety incidents.*

Henriksen K, Battles JB, Marks ES, et al., editors. *Advances in Patient Safety: From Research to Implementation* (Volume 4: Programs, Tools, and Products). Rockville (MD): Agency for Healthcare Research and Quality (US); February 2005.

GPhC. *Guidance on raising concerns.* (**www.pharmacyregulation.org**) (see Appendix 6)

RPS. *Raising concerns, whistle blowing and speaking up safely in Pharmacy.* September 2011. (**www.rpharms.com/resources-AtoZ**)

RPS. *8 core principles for community pharmacy whistle blowing policies and procedures.* September 2011. (**www.rpharms.com/resources-AtoZ**)

RPS. *The speaking up charter.* 2012. (**www.rpharms.com**)

Leonard M, Frankel A. *How can leaders influence a safety culture? The Health Foundation;* May 2012. (**www.health.org.uk**)

National Patient Safety Agency. *Seven steps to patient safety: A guide for NHS staff.* July 2014 (**www.nrls.npsa.nhs.uk**)

PharmacyQS.com. *10 Improvement challenges: improve culture.* (**www.pharmacyqs.com**)

RPS. *Leadership development framework and accompanying handbook.* (**www.rpharms.com**)

NHS Improvement. *Freedom to speak up: raising concerns (whistleblowing) policy for the NHS.* April 2016. (**https://improvement.nhs.uk/resources/**)

START HERE

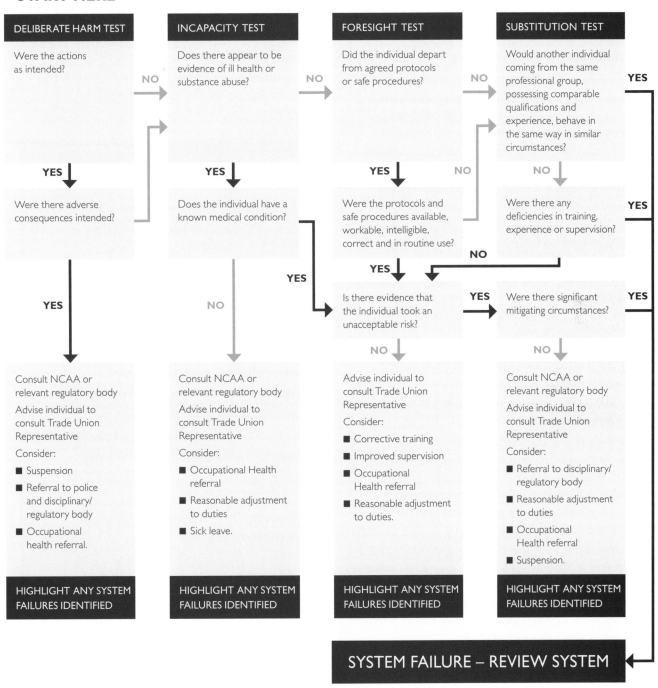

DELIBERATE HARM TEST

Were the actions as intended?

NO →

YES ↓

Were there adverse consequences intended?

YES ↓

Consult NCAA or relevant regulatory body

Advise individual to consult Trade Union Representative

Consider:

■ Suspension
■ Referral to police and disciplinary/ regulatory body
■ Occupational health referral.

HIGHLIGHT ANY SYSTEM FAILURES IDENTIFIED

INCAPACITY TEST

Does there appear to be evidence of ill health or substance abuse?

NO →

YES ↓

Does the individual have a known medical condition?

NO ↓

Consult NCAA or relevant regulatory body

Advise individual to consult Trade Union Representative

Consider:

■ Occupational Health referral
■ Reasonable adjustment to duties
■ Sick leave.

HIGHLIGHT ANY SYSTEM FAILURES IDENTIFIED

FORESIGHT TEST

Did the individual depart from agreed protocols or safe procedures?

NO →

YES ↓   NO

Were the protocols and safe procedures available, workable, intelligible, correct and in routine use?

YES ↓

Is there evidence that the individual took an unacceptable risk?   **YES** →

NO ↓

Advise individual to consult Trade Union Representative

Consider:

■ Corrective training
■ Improved supervision
■ Occupational Health referral
■ Reasonable adjustment to duties.

HIGHLIGHT ANY SYSTEM FAILURES IDENTIFIED

SUBSTITUTION TEST

Would another individual coming from the same professional group, possessing comparable qualifications and experience, behave in the same way in similar circumstances?

NO →   **YES**

NO ↓

Were there any deficiencies in training, experience or supervision?   **YES**

NO

Were there significant mitigating circumstances?   **YES**

NO ↓

Consult NCAA or relevant regulatory body

Advise individual to consult Trade Union Representative

Consider:

■ Referral to disciplinary/ regulatory body
■ Reasonable adjustment to duties
■ Occupational Health referral
■ Suspension.

HIGHLIGHT ANY SYSTEM FAILURES IDENTIFIED

SYSTEM FAILURE – REVIEW SYSTEM ←

DIAGRAM 4: REPRODUCTION OF THE NHS INCIDENT DECISION TREE

We have included the NHS incident decision tree which is subject to Crown copyright and reproduced under the terms of the Open Government Licence as an illustration of a process which is fair and balances learning and accountability.

NCAA stands for National Clinical Assessment Authority and became part of the National Clinical Assessment Service (NCAS).

2.7 Professional empowerment

Professional empowerment is about enabling professionalism.

At an individual level for pharmacists and future pharmacists, it is about the development of knowledge; development of skills, experience and confidence; and the cultivation of professional values and behaviours which collectively imbue the pharmacist with authority, empowering and enabling professionalism.

At a wider level it is about creating an environment around an individual which enables all of the above.

Professional training starts at university and is enhanced with pre-registration training by learning, pre-registration tutors and training programmes. In professional practice it is self-cultivated through *continuing professional development (CPD)* (see section 2.8.1) and continuing education, and supported by pharmacy organisations through training programmes and events.

The General Pharmaceutical Council (GPhC) standards for registered pharmacies require that *Staff are empowered and competent to safeguard the health, safety and wellbeing of patients and the public* (see Appendix 2 for further information).

The Royal Pharmaceutical Society contributes to creating empowerment through guidance, standards, news and alerts; through webinars and our mentoring programme; through our Leadership Development Framework; through influencing policy and embedding and nurturing the *right culture* (see section 2.6).

Employers play a key role by providing structured training resources and events; conferences; opportunity and time for CPD; support from the superintendent or office of the superintendent; company alerts and updates; developing and implementing the right organisation culture which enables professional empowerment.

Other pharmacy organisations, stakeholders and training providers are also integral to enabling professionalism through training, and enabling the right environment for professionalism to flourish, including through getting the culture right.

FURTHER RESOURCES

RPS. *Leadership development framework and accompanying handbook.* **(www.rpharms.com)**

RPS. *Reducing workplace pressure through professional empowerment.* (July 2011). **(www.rpharms.com/professional-empowerment/member-resources.asp)**

RPS. *Employing a locum.* **(www.rpharms.com/professional-empowerment/member-resources.asp)**

RPS. *Locums: Working as a Responsible Pharmacist.* **(www.rpharms.com/professional-empowerment/member-resources.asp)**

RPS. *Locum pharmacists: Working as a locum pharmacist in community quick reference guide.* (December 2013). **(www.rpharms.com/resources-AtoZ)**

2.8 Professional development

2.8.1 CONTINUING PROFESSIONAL DEVELOPMENT (CPD)

2.8.2 RPS FACULTY

2.8.3 RPS FOUNDATION PROGRAMME

2.8.4 DEVELOPING LEADERSHIP

2.8.5 MENTORING

Learning and the development of skills and expertise is important for all pharmacists at any stage of their career. Keeping up to date with the relevant knowledge and skills will help you practise safely and confidently.

The following RPS resources can help you with your professional development at any stage of your career. Detailed information on each of the following can be found on the RPS website at: **www.rpharms.com/ development/continuing-professional-development.asp**

2.8.1 CONTINUING PROFESSIONAL DEVELOPMENT (CPD)

There is a statutory requirement for pharmacists to record their CPD. You must make a minimum of nine CPD entries per registration year. The criteria for the review of CPD records require you to submit nine entries completed for each full review period with three of these starting at the reflection phase of the CPD cycle. The entries must be relevant to the safe and effective practice of pharmacy and your own scope of practice.

The GPhC specifies that your entries submitted should follow the GPhC CPD cycle. The cycle consists of the following four phased learning process:

- **REFLECTION** – thinking about your practice as a pharmacist
- **PLANNING** – deciding how and when you are going to learn, what you want to learn to do
- **ACTION** – recording what you learnt
- **EVALUATION** – identifying the benefits of your learning.

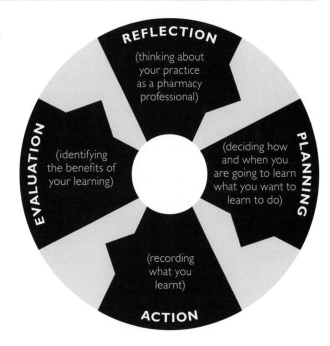

DIAGRAM 5: THE GPhC CPD CYCLE

2.8.2 RPS FACULTY

The RPS Faculty is the pharmacy professional recognition programme for RPS members which provides you with a way of identifying what you need to know at different levels of practice, across all sectors. It allows you to advance as a specialist or generalist and recognise your development thereby demonstrating to colleagues, healthcare professionals, patients and the public your advanced or specialised level of practice through the award and use of post nominals. The Faculty is for RPS members who have completed their early years of practice.

2.8.3 RPS FOUNDATION PROGRAMME

Foundation Practice is the knowledge, skills and behaviours that collectively form the building blocks for all pharmacists across all sectors. We know that pharmacy practitioners who are well supported and understand what is required are better equipped to adapt and deliver pharmaceutical care. The Foundation Pharmacy Framework (FPF) provides a structured approach to paving the way for you to realise your competence, demonstrate your experience, facilitate advancement or develop special interests.

The Foundation Programme is an integrated workforce development that aims to provide access to support for practitioners from recently qualified to those who are returning to work after career breaks, and to those who may be changing their scope of practice or practice environment or simply working steadily.

2.8.4 DEVELOPING LEADERSHIP

The Leadership Development Framework applies to all pharmacy professionals at every stage of their professional journey; from the time they enter formal training, become qualified as a practitioner and throughout their continuing professional development as experienced practitioners.

The Leadership Development Framework is based on the concept of engaging, collective leadership for all, whether in a leadership role or not. It promotes leadership behaviours (the 'how-to-do' of leadership) across all sectors of the profession and encourages a collective responsibility for the success of an organisation and its services. Engaging leadership can come from anyone in an organisation, as appropriate, and at different times, and is an essential element of good practice and professional development.

2.8.5 MENTORING

The RPS mentoring service enables pharmacists practising at every level in all sectors of pharmacy to benefit from the support and guidance of their more experienced colleagues through a variety of approaches to mentoring.

The RPS online mentor-mentee database allows you to access a mentor to suit your needs or to volunteer your services as a mentor. We also help you to link up with other members of your profession for both offering and receiving mentoring support through local practice forums, RPS professional support, online groups and our website.

2.9 Research involvement

Pharmacists, regardless of their workplace setting, are becoming increasingly involved in research activities. For some pharmacists, particularly those working in industry and academia, research will be a major part of their role. It is important that pharmacists have a good understanding of the ethical implications and requirements for research and how these impact on their working practices. This applies whether they are leading the research themselves or being asked to participate in research led by others – research is often a multidisciplinary team activity. For both of these types of involvement pharmacists can seek advice from a range of sources. The General Pharmaceutical Council's seven principles within the *Standards of conduct, ethics and performance* (see Appendix 1) apply to research just as they do to any other area of pharmacy practice. Examples of how they apply to research are provided below:

1. **Make patients your first concern** – Is the research relevant to your patient/service user population? Does the research have the necessary approvals (Ethics, NHS R&D)? Consider the harm and benefit of the research to patients, carers and/or the public and protect their health, safety and wellbeing.

2. **Use your professional judgement in the interests of patients and public** – Who is proposing the research? are there any areas for potential conflict of interest?

3. **Show respect for others** – Respect and protect participant confidentiality, respect individuals' decisions if they chose not to participate, maintain confidentiality, respect all other colleagues involved in the research.

4. **Encourage patients and the public to participate in decisions about their care** – Ensure participants are fully informed about the research and their consent to participate is freely given. Where possible, encourage patients, their carers and the public to get involved in the design of the research and its dissemination.

5. **Develop your professional knowledge and competence** – Pharmacists need to understand the reasons for doing the research. Pharmacists should follow the study guidance or protocol exactly to ensure consistency of delivery of an intervention or data collection from different sites. They must be competent or seek training in all areas of the research in which they are involved. Ensure adherence to the law relating to privacy and confidentiality, e.g. Data Protection Act.

6. **Be honest and trustworthy** – Maintain accurate records, ensure all recruited patients are eligible, do not falsify results or exclude 'negative' findings.

7. **Take responsibility for your working practices** – Pharmacists should take responsibility for their level of participation within the research, i.e. you are responsible for the area of research you are involved in, such as the length of time and activities involved. Does your pharmacy have the appropriate resources to conduct the research?

GENERAL POINTS FOR CONSIDERATION

ABOUT THE RESEARCH

- Who is conducting the research?
- Is the purpose of the research clear?
- Is there potential harm/benefit to participants?
- Has the study been granted ethical approval through an NHS research ethics committee or another appropriate organisation?
- Is the study relevant to you and/or your patients, carers or the public?
- Has participant consent been addressed?
- Will all participants be informed of the results?

ABOUT YOUR INVOLVEMENT

- Are you clear about your role in the study?
- Do you have the appropriate resources (staff and facilities) to accommodate the research?
- Do you have the relevant skills or do you require training?
- Is participant confidentiality assured?
- Where and how is data being stored?
- Is data transfer to a third party secure and appropriate?

FURTHER READING AND SOURCES OF ADVICE

RPS. *Science and research.* **(www.rpharms.com/research)**

RPS. *Local practice forums.* **(www.rpharms.com)** *(GB wide)*

RPS. *Research ready guidance.* **(www.rpharms.com/researchready)** *(UK wide)*

The Health Research Authority. (www.hra.nhs.uk) *(UK wide)*

Local NHS Research and Development Offices. (www.rdforum.nhs.uk) *(UK wide)*

Research Design Services *(England).* **(www.rds.nihr.ac.uk)**

Research Design Services *(Wales).* **(http://www.healthandcareresearch.gov.wales/ research-design-and-conduct-service/)**

The Integrated Research Application System. (www.myresearchproject.org.uk) *(UK wide)*

Local Schools of Pharmacy

National Institute for Health Research. *Ok to ask.* **(http://www.nihr.ac.uk/get-involved/ ok-to-ask.htm)**

3. UNDERPINNING KNOWLEDGE – LEGISLATION AND PROFESSIONAL ISSUES

The exercise of professional judgement by a pharmacist is underpinned by relevant knowledge. Components of this knowledge are an awareness of pharmacy legislation, professional standards and good practice.

The Human Medicines Regulations 2012 consolidated most of the legislation regulating the authorisation, sale and supply of medicinal products for human use, made under the Medicines Act 1968. It is important to understand that the Medicines Act 1968 has not been replaced fully and that certain parts are still active. Further information on the Human Medicines Regulations 2012 and the consolidation can be found in Chapter 2 of Dale and Appelbe's Pharmacy and Medicines Law (10th Edition) and the MHRA website **www.gov.uk/government/organisations/medicines-and-healthcare-products-regulatory-agency** (search for 'Human Medicines Regulations 2012').

The Veterinary Medicines Regulations, last updated in 2013, covers the prescribing and supply for animals. The first VMR came into force in 2005, to consolidate controls on veterinary medicines which had historically been part of the Medicines Act 1968. Further information on the Veterinary Medicines Regulations can be found in Chapter 16 of Dale and Appelbe's Pharmacy and Medicines Law (10th Edition) and the Veterinary Medicines Directorate (VMD) website at **www.gov.uk/government/organisations/veterinary-medicines-directorate** (search for 'Veterinary Medicines Regulations').

The Programme Board for Rebalancing Medicines Legislation and Pharmacy Regulation reviews relevant pharmacy legislation and regulation to ensure it provides safety for users of pharmacy services. It facilitates a systematic approach to quality in pharmacy, allowing innovation and development of pharmacy practice, whilst reducing the burden of unnecessary and inflexible regulations. The Programme will build on and propose amendments to legislation as required, to deliver a modern approach to regulation which maintains patient and public safety, whilst supporting professional and quality systems development, including learning from dispensing errors made in registered pharmacies.

Further information and updates on the Rebalancing Medicines Legislation and Pharmacy Regulation Programme Board can be found on the RPS website at **www.rpharms.com/political-issues/rebalancing-legislation.asp** and on the UK government website at **www.gov.uk/government/groups/pharmacy-regulation-programme-board.**

The MEP is not intended to be a complete repository of pharmacy legislation and aims instead to provide a practical resource, professional guide and digest to the most relevant aspects of pharmacy legislation.

3.1 Classification of medicines

Pharmacists deal with three classes of medicinal products for humans under the Human Medicines Regulations 2012 and several classes of veterinary medicinal products under the Veterinary Medicines Regulations. An understanding of these and associated professional issues is important to pharmacists as medicines should not be considered normal items of commerce, and the final decision on sale or supply is one determined by the professional judgement of the pharmacist.

Pharmacists are empowered to refuse to sell or supply ANY medicines, if the sale or supply is contrary to the pharmacist's clinical judgement.

There will be different situations requiring varying levels of explanation as to why a sale or supply was refused. This will depend upon whether or not it is the patient who is asking and if not whether the person asking has clinical expertise and a legitimate interest.

General sale medicines

General sale medicines (commonly known as GSL medicines) are those that can be sold in registered pharmacies but also in other retail outlets that can 'close so as to exclude the public'. They are classified as general sale medicines mostly because of an EU or UK marketing authorisation (product licence), if they hold a traditional herbal registration or if they have a certificate of registration as a general sale medicine homeopathic product.

The term (PO) medicine is sometimes used by manufacturers as a term that describes a product that is licensed as a general sale medicine but for which the manufacturer wishes to restrict sales or supplies through pharmacies only (e.g. 30-sachet packs of Fybogel).

Within a pharmacy, general sale medicines can only be sold when a pharmacist has assumed the role of responsible pharmacist; however, the pharmacist may be physically absent for a limited period of time while remaining responsible, thus permitting sales of general sale medicines during this absence (see Appendix 10).

Pharmacy (P) medicines

A pharmacy medicine is a medicinal product that can be sold from a registered pharmacy premises by a pharmacist or a person acting under the supervision of a pharmacist.

Together with general sale medicines, P medicines are collectively known as over-the-counter (OTC) or non-prescription medicines. The sale of some of these medicines is associated with additional legal and professional considerations; the most common issues are explained in section 3.2.

SELF-SELECTION OF P MEDICINES

The General Pharmaceutical Council at its 13 September 2012 meeting made it clear that the self-selection of P medicines is prohibited until they are able to enforce standards for registered pharmacies and that a further additional regulatory pre-condition around self selection is that guidance on compliance in this area would need to have been developed and communicated in advance of any change.

In addition to the regulatory standards outlined above, our interim statement of professional standard for the supply of OTC medicines also references self-selection and states that *Pharmacy medicines must not be accessible to the public by self selection*. For up-to-date information on self selection of P medicines and a full copy of the interim statement see our website at **www.rpharms.com/support-resources/support-resources-a-z.asp**.

Prescription-only medicines (POM)

A prescription-only medicine (POM) is a medicine that is generally subject to the restriction of requiring a prescription written by an appropriate practitioner: doctor, dentist, supplementary prescriber, nurse independent prescriber, pharmacist independent prescriber, EEA and Swiss doctors and dentists (but not for all Controlled Drugs), EEA and Swiss prescribing pharmacist and prescribing nurse where they exist, community practitioner nurses (for a limited selection of POMs), optometrist independent prescribers (not for

Controlled Drugs, or parenteral medicines), podiatrist, physiotherapist and therapeutic radiographer independent prescribers (for certain medicines see section 3.3.1) before it can be sold or supplied. There are exemptions to requiring a prescription in some circumstances (see section 3.3.10). Further details about the legal and professional issues associated with POMs are discussed in section 3.3.

Some medicines can be classified under more than one category and this can depend upon formulation, strength, quantity, indication or marketing authorisation.

FURTHER RESOURCES

Appelbe GE, Wingfield J, editors. *Dale and Applebe's Pharmacy and Medicines Law.* 10th edition. London: Pharmaceutical Press; 2013.

An A-Z list of medicines for human use and their legal classification is available to members on the Royal Pharmaceutical Society website **(www.rpharms.com) (Please see disclaimer on the website when using this list).**

3.2 Professional and legal issues: pharmacy medicines

3.2.1 PSEUDOEPHEDRINE AND EPHEDRINE

3.2.2 ORAL EMERGENCY CONTRACEPTIVES AS PHARMACY MEDICINES

3.2.3 PARACETAMOL AND ASPIRIN

3.2.4 CODEINE AND DIHYDROCODEINE

3.2.5 COUGH AND COLD MEDICINES FOR CHILDREN

3.2.6 RECLASSIFIED MEDICINES

3.2.1 PSEUDOEPHEDRINE AND EPHEDRINE

Pseudoephedrine and ephedrine are widely used decongestant pharmacy medicines. However, due to their potential for misuse in the illicit production of methylamphetamine (crystal meth) – a class A Controlled Drug – there are legal restrictions on the quantities that can be sold or supplied without prescription. A class A drug is associated with the most severe penalties for possession and dealing.

■ It is unlawful to supply a product or combination of products that contain more than 720mg of pseudoephedrine OR 180mg of ephedrine at any one time, without a prescription (Regulation 237 of Human Medicines Regulations 2012)

■ It is unlawful to sell or supply any pseudoephedrine product at the same time as an ephedrine product without a prescription (Regulation 237 of Human Medicines Regulations 2012).

SIGNS OF POSSIBLE MISUSE

The following signs in combination can be useful for identifying when a request is more likely to be suspicious:

■ **NERVOUS OR GUILTY BEHAVIOUR** – avoiding eye contact, appearing to be uncomfortable answering questions, unusually timid

■ **LACK OF SYMPTOMS** – not suffering from cough, cold or flu symptoms, or unable to describe these in the patient if buying for someone else

■ **REHEARSED ANSWERS** – gives answers that appear to be rehearsed or scripted

■ **IMPATIENT OR AGGRESSIVE** – in a rush or hurrying to complete the transaction

■ **OPPORTUNISTIC** – waiting for busy periods in the shop or until less experienced staff are available

■ **SPECIFIC PRODUCTS** – wants certain brands that contain only pseudoephedrine or ephedrine

■ **PARAPHERNALIA** – wishes also to purchase other items which can be used to manufacture methylamphetamine (e.g. lithium batteries, chemicals such as acetone)

■ **QUANTITIES** – requests large quantities

■ **FREQUENCY** – makes frequent requests.

Sales or supplies of pseudoephedrine or ephedrine should either be made personally by the pharmacist or by pharmacy staff who have been trained and are competent to deal with pseudoephedrine and ephedrine issues, and who know when it is necessary to refer to the pharmacist.

Even when a request is made for a lawful quantity, the sale or supply can be refused where there are reasonable grounds for suspecting misuse. A person purchasing pseudoephedrine and ephedrine for illicit purposes may not be a 'user' of methylamphetamine and, therefore, may not conform to stereotypes. They may be male, female and of any age or background.

Suspicions can be reported to your local GPhC inspector, local Controlled Drugs liaison police officer or accountable officer.

FURTHER READING

RPS. *Pseudoephedrine and ephedrine – quick reference guide.* 2010. (www.rpharms.com/resources-AtoZ)

3.2.2 ORAL EMERGENCY CONTRACEPTIVES AS PHARMACY MEDICINES

Levonorgestrel 1500 microgram tablet and ulipristal acetate 30mg tablet are licensed as pharmacy medicines for emergency hormonal contraception (EHC). Levonorgestrel is licensed as a pharmacy medicine for women aged 16 years or over for emergency contraception within 72 hours of unprotected sexual intercourse or failure of a contraceptive method. Ulipristal acetate is licensed for emergency contraception within 120 hours (5 days) of unprotected sexual intercourse or failure of a contraceptive method. The pharmacist should be involved in assessing suitability and approving sales.

Advance supply of oral EHC

Pharmacists can provide an advance supply of oral emergency contraception (i.e. prior to unprotected sexual intercourse or in case of failure of a contraceptive method) to a patient requesting it at a pharmacy. The patient should be assessed to ensure that they are competent, they intend to use the medicine appropriately and it is clinically appropriate.

Religious or moral beliefs

See Appendix 8 for provisional GPhC guidance on the provision of pharmacy services affected by religious or moral beliefs.

Vulnerable adults and children

Be aware that, in some circumstances, requests for EHC could be linked to abuse (non-consensual intercourse) of children or vulnerable adults. The Department of Health has published a document called *Responding to domestic abuse: A handbook for health professionals*, which provides practical advice on dealing with domestic abuse, keeping records, confidentiality and sharing information.

The Department for Education has published a guidance document called *Working together to safeguard children*, which includes sections for health professionals and on referral.

The supply of ulipristal acetate to patients under the age of 16 years is not contraindicated by the manufacturer, however pharmacists may wish to consider the following additional factors:

- Children under the age of 13 are legally too young to consent to any sexual activity. Instances should be treated seriously with a presumption that the case should be reported to social services, unless there are exceptional circumstances backed by documented reasons for not sharing information

- Sexual activity with children under the age of 16 is also an offence but may be consensual. The law is not intended to prosecute mutually agreed sexual activity between young people of a similar age, unless it involves abuse or exploitation

■ Pharmacists can provide contraception or sexual health advice to a child under the age of 16 and the general duty of patient confidentiality applies, so where there is a decision to share information consent should be sought whenever possible prior to disclosing patient information. This duty is not absolute and information may be shared if you judge on a case-by-case basis that sharing is in the child's best interest (e.g. to prevent harm to the child or where the child's welfare overrides the need to keep information confidential). Remember that it is possible to seek advice from experts without disclosing identifiable details of a child and breaking patient confidentiality – and that where there is a decision to share information, this should be proportionate.

Other mechanisms for supply

There are various mechanisms for the supply of EHC and it may be appropriate to refer to other service providers rather than make a sale, in some circumstances (e.g. where a sale would be outside of the terms of the marketing authorisation). Other providers include family planning clinics, general practice clinics and providers of PGDs for EHC and genitourinary medicine (GUM) clinics.

The quick reference guide *Oral Emergency Contraceptives as Pharmacy Medicines* can be used to obtain relevant information to determine whether supply is appropriate or not. The guidance also includes advice that can be given to a patient after a supply has been made. It is available on the RPS website at: **www.rpharms.com/resources-AtoZ**

FURTHER READING

RPS. *Oral emergency contraceptives as pharmacy medicines – quick reference guide.* 2015. **(www.rpharms.com/resources-AtoZ)**

Online resources are available from the Faculty of Sexual & Reproductive Healthcare website **(www.fsrh.org)**

Department for Education. *Working together to safeguard children.* March 2015. **(www.gov.uk/government/organisations/department-for-education)**

Faculty of Sexual & Reproductive Healthcare. *A quality standard for contraceptive services.* March 2014. **(www.fsrh.org)**

NICE. *Contraceptive services for under 25s (PH51).* March 2014. **(www.nice.org.uk)**

Online resources are available from the National Society for the Prevention of Cruelty to Children website **(www.nspcc.org.uk)**. The society also has a helpline (Tel: 0808 800 5000)

Department of Health (National Archives). *Responding to domestic abuse: A handbook for health professionals.* December 2005. **(http://webarchive. nationalarchives.gov.uk/20060123125814/dh.gov. uk/en/publicationsandstatistics/publications/ publicationspolicyandguidance/dh_4126161)**

Centre for Pharmacy Postgraduate Education. *Emergency contraception.* **(www.cppe.ac.uk)**

Wales Centre for Pharmacy Postgraduate Education. *Emergency contraception.* **(www.wcppe.org.uk)**

NHS Education for Scotland. *Contraception.* **(www.nes.scot.nhs.uk/)**

Department of Health (National Archives). *Best practice guidance for doctors and other health professionals on the provision of advice and treatment to young people under 16 on contraception, sexual and reproductive health.* 2004. **(http://webarchive. nationalarchives.gov.uk/+/www.dh.gov.uk/ en/Publicationsandstatistics/Publications/ publicationspolicyandguidance/DH_4086960)**

Scottish Government. *National Guidance. Under-age sexual activity: meeting the needs of children and young people and identifying child protection concerns.* 2010. **(www.gov.scot)**

Family Planning Association. *Law on sex factsheet.* 2015. **(www.fpa.org.uk)**

GPhC. *Guidance on patient confidentiality.* See Appendix 4 or www.pharmacyregulation.org

GPhC. *Guidance on Consent.* See Appendix 5 or www.pharmacyregulation.org

3.2.3 PARACETAMOL AND ASPIRIN

Paracetamol and aspirin are medicinal products that are available in a range of formulations, strengths and packaged quantities. They have marketing authorisations as POM, P and general sale medicines – depending upon pack size and formulation. Legal restrictions on the total quantities of certain formulations of these medicines that can be sold without prescription have been deemed necessary. Table 1 illustrates the quantities of paracetamol and aspirin that can be sold legally.

TABLE 1: PARACETAMOL AND ASPIRIN – OTC LEGAL RESTRICTIONS

	LEGAL RESTRICTION	ADDITIONAL NOTE
PARACETAMOL	Not more than 100 non-effervescent* tablets or capsules can be sold to a person at any one time. Since most OTC pack sizes are for 16 or 32 dose units, this means that, in practice, less than 100 non-effervescent tablets or capsules can be sold.	There are no legal limits on the quantity of over-the-counter effervescent* tablets, powders, granules or liquids that can be sold to a person at any one time. Use professional judgement to decide the appropriate quantity to supply and what limits to impose.
ASPIRIN	Not more than 100 non-effervescent* tablets or capsules can be sold to a person at any one time. Since most OTC pack sizes are for 16 or 32 dose units, this means that, in practice, less than 100 non-effervescent tablets or capsules can be sold.	There are no legal limits on the quantities of over-the-counter effervescent* tablets or powders that can be sold to a person at any one time. Use professional judgement to decide the appropriate quantity to supply and what limits to impose.

NB: The definition of effervescent for the purposes of the restrictions above is provided by medicines legislation. Soluble or dispersible formulations as defined by the British Pharmacopoeia may not meet the definition of effervescent in medicines legislation. Where in doubt, quantities of soluble or dispersible formulations sold should be restricted as non-effervescent preparations.

FURTHER READING

RPS. *PSB 9: Supplying over-the-counter analgesics.* January 2012. (**www.rpharms.com**)

3.2.4 CODEINE AND DIHYDROCODEINE

In September 2009, the Medicines and Healthcare products Regulatory Agency (MHRA) announced that there would be tighter controls and new warnings on packaging of OTC solid dose medicines (e.g. tablets and capsules) containing codeine or dihydrocodeine. These were introduced to minimise the risk of overuse and addiction of these medicines.

The necessary changes to marketing authorisations (product licences) for pre-existing OTC codeine and dihydrocodeine medicines were completed by 31 December 2009. From the date that the marketing authorisation was changed, all new batches would have been manufactured and labelled with the new warnings and subject to the tighter controls.

The changes include:

- **INDICATIONS** – indications for solid dose OTC codeine and dihydrocodeine products are now restricted to the short-term treatment of acute, moderate pain that is not relieved by paracetamol, ibuprofen or aspirin alone. All other previous indications, including cold, flu, cough, sore throats and minor pain have been removed

- **PACK SIZES** – any pack containing more than 32 dose units now requires a marketing authorisation as a POM. This includes effervescent formulations

- **PILLS AND LABELS** – the warning 'Can cause addiction. For three days use only' must now be positioned in a prominent clear position on the front of the pack. In addition, both the PIL and packaging need to state the indication and that the medicine can cause addiction or overuse headache if used continuously for more than three days. The PIL must also contain information about the warning signs of addiction.

The RPS supports the purpose of these tighter controls and recommends that only one pack of OTC medication containing codeine or dihydrocodeine should be sold, as sale of more than one pack would undermine the reduction in pack size and POM restriction on packs containing more than 32 dose units.

Updated packaging and product information will have been available since June 2010.

3.2.5 COUGH AND COLD MEDICINES FOR CHILDREN

In 2009 the Commission on Human Medicines reviewed the evidence for using cough and cold medicines in children and found that there were limited studies to support this use. These medicines had been introduced in the past when requirements to demonstrate safety and efficacy were less demanding than they were in 2009.

As a result, the MHRA issued important advice affecting the use of cough and cold medicines in children aged below 12, which resulted in significant changes to the marketing authorisations for these medicines.

Many cough and cold medicines are no longer used in children under six years of age as there is no evidence that they are effective and, in some cases, the ingredients are linked to side effects including allergies, sleep disturbances and hallucinations.

Medicines containing the following ingredients have been deemed unsuitable for children under 6 years:

- **ANTITUSSIVES** – dextromethorphan, pholcodine
- **EXPECTORANTS** – guaifenesin, ipecacuanha
- **NASAL DECONGESTANTS** – ephedrine, oxymetazoline, phenylephrine, pseudoephedrine, xylometazoline
- **ANTIHISTAMINES** – brompheniramine, chlorphenamine, diphenhydramine, doxylamine, promethazine, triprolidine.

Cough and cold medicines for children aged 6-12 years containing the above ingredients are now indicated for use as second line to best practice (see overleaf) and should not be used for more than five days. Warning labels on the packaging and labelling for these medicines have been strengthened to reflect the 2009 advice.

There is also an ongoing change to ensure that all liquid cough and cold medicines are supplied in a child-resistant container.

Useful lists (non-exhaustive) of the medicinal products that can be sold or supplied for use by children under six years of age, and for children aged between six and 12 years, are available on the RPS website (**www.rpharms.com/resources-AtoZ**).

Best practice for treating children with a cough and/or a cold

Most colds will resolve within five to seven days. However, the following treatment or advice can be given as first-line remedies if the symptoms are causing discomfort or distress. All medicines must also be given in accordance with licensed indications:

- **FOR ALL SYMPTOMS** – non-pharmacological interventions such as advising that the child drinks plenty of fluids
- **FOR FEVER AND PAIN** – treat with paracetamol or ibuprofen. National Institute for Health and Clinical Excellence (NICE) guidelines (**www.nice.org.uk**) do not currently recommend using paracetamol and ibuprofen at the same time in children under five years. Currently, the second of these medicines should only be considered if the child does not respond to the first
- **FOR NASAL CONGESTION** – treat with saline nasal drops, vapour rubs or decongestants, or steam inhalation
- **FOR A COUGH** – warm, clear fluids or warm lemon and honey drinks can be advised if the child is aged over one year. Also, simple cough mixtures such as glycerol or simple linctus can be recommended.

If symptoms persist or you suspect that it may be a more serious condition, refer the patient to their GP.

Sale of medicines containing the listed ingredients for indications other than cough and cold

Medicines containing those ingredients listed above can continue to be sold for use in children for licensed indications other than cough and cold. For example, Piriton (chlorpheniramine) is not licensed for treating a cough or cold so should not be sold for this purpose. However, it can be sold for its licensed uses.

Codeine linctus for dry, unproductive coughs in children and young people

The MHRA issued new advice in October 2010 that OTC liquid preparations containing codeine should not be used in children or young people under 18 years because the risks outweigh the benefits. This affected all codeine linctus BP products that were licensed at the time for use in those under 18 years (including Pulmo Bailly, Galcodine linctus and Galcodine paediatric linctus).

FURTHER READING

Department of Health (National Archives). *Birth to Five* (2009 edition). (**http://webarchive. nationalarchives.gov.uk/20130107105354/http:// dh.gov.uk/health/category/publications/**)

Online resources are available on the NHS Choices website (**www.nhs.uk**)

RPS. *Children's cough and cold – quick reference guide.* 2010. (**www.rpharms.com/resources-AtoZ**)

Online resources are available on the MHRA website (**www.gov.uk/government/organisations/ medicines-and-healthcare-products-regulatory- agency**)

NICE. *Feverish illness in children: Assessment and initial management in children younger than 5 years.* May 2013. (**www.nice.org.uk**)

3.2.6 RECLASSIFIED MEDICINES

Increasingly, more medicines are being reclassified from POM to P, providing pharmacists with a larger repertoire of medicines to select from to treat patients. It is appropriate that pharmacists involved in the sale of reclassified medicines are appropriately trained on relevant clinical and best practice aspects of the medicines and that pharmacy support staff are trained and/or work under protocols (as appropriate) when they supply these medicines. This is particularly relevant to newly reclassified POM to P medicines but also applies to all reclassifications and P medicines generally.

FURTHER RESOURCES

Guidance for the following reclassified medicines is available from the RPS website (**www.rpharms.com**; search for 'Reclassifications'):

Amorolfine nail lacquer

Azithromycin

Chloramphenicol eye drops and eye ointment

Levonorgestrel and ulipristal acetate (see oral emergency contraceptives as pharmacy medicines)

Omeprazole

Orlistat

Sumatriptan

Tamsulosin

Tranexamic acid

UNDERPINNING KNOWLEDGE – LEGISLATION AND PROFESSIONAL ISSUES

3.3 Professional and legal issues: prescription-only medicines

3.3.1   GENERAL PRESCRIPTION REQUIREMENTS

3.3.2   FAXED PRESCRIPTIONS

3.3.3   DENTAL PRESCRIPTIONS

3.3.4   FORGED PRESCRIPTIONS

3.3.5   PRESCRIPTIONS FROM THE EEA OR SWITZERLAND

3.3.6   MILITARY PRESCRIPTIONS

3.3.7   LABELLING OF DISPENSED MEDICINAL PRODUCTS

3.3.8   ADMINISTRATION

3.3.9   PATIENT SPECIFIC DIRECTIONS AND ADMINISTRATION, SALE OR SUPPLY IN HOSPITALS AND OTHER SETTINGS

3.3.10 EXEMPTIONS: SALE AND SUPPLY WITHOUT A PRESCRIPTION

3.3.11 SELF-PRESCRIBED PRESCRIPTIONS AND PRESCRIPTIONS FOR CLOSE FRIENDS AND FAMILY

3.3.12 SUPPLYING ISOTRETINOIN AND PREGNANCY PREVENTION

3.3.13 DISPENSING VALPROATE FOR GIRLS AND WOMEN

3.3.14 EXPLAINING BIOSIMILAR MEDICINES

3.3.15 SUMMARY OF PRESCRIBER TYPES AND PRESCRIBING RESTRICTIONS

3.3.16 CHECKING REGISTRATION OF HEALTHCARE PROFESSIONALS AND ADDITIONAL INFORMATION ON CONDITIONS OF SUPPLY

3.3.1 GENERAL PRESCRIPTION REQUIREMENTS

The sale, supply and administration of prescription-only medicines (POMs) are restricted by the Human Medicines Regulations 2012. The main routes by which a pharmacist is able to sell or supply a POM is under the authority of a prescription from an appropriate practitioner (for example, a doctor, dentist, supplementary prescriber, independent prescriber or community practitioner nurse), or via an exemption (see section 3.3.10). Further information on different types of appropriate practitioner, prescribing restrictions and checking registration can be found in sections 3.3.15 and 3.3.16.

Information on requirements for prescriptions issued by prescribers registered in an EEA country or Switzerland can be found in section 3.3.5.

NB: The additional prescription requirements for Controlled Drugs are discussed in section 3.7.7.

Several pieces of information must be present for a prescription to be legal (Regulation 217 and 218 Human Medicines Regulations 2012). These are specified in Diagram 6.

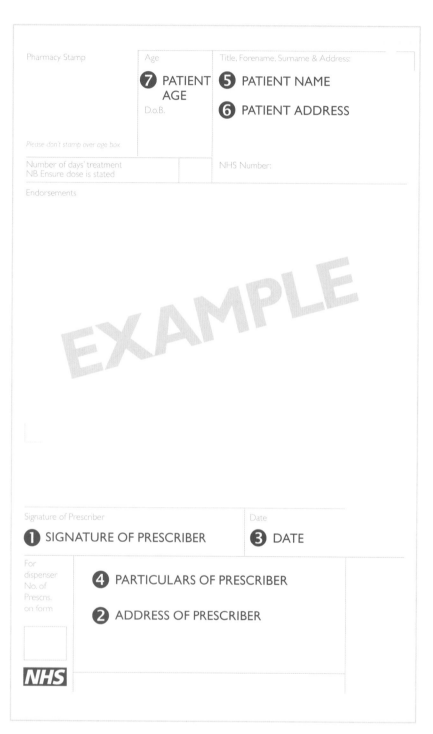

1 SIGNATURE – prescriptions need to be signed in ink by an appropriate practitioner (see sections 3.3.1 and 3.3.14) in his or her own name. An 'advanced electronic signature' can be used to authorise an electronic prescription (see blue box on next page for further information).

2 ADDRESS – prescriptions must include the address of the appropriate practitioner (see 3.3.1).

3 DATE – a prescription is valid for up to six months from the *appropriate* date (for prescriptions for Schedules 2, 3 or 4 Controlled Drugs, see section 3.7.7). For an NHS prescription, the appropriate date is the later of either the date on which the prescription was signed or a date indicated by the appropriate practitioner as the date before which it should not be dispensed. For private prescriptions, the appropriate date will always be the date on which it was signed.

4 PARTICULARS – prescriptions require particulars that indicate the type of appropriate practitioner (see section 3.3.1).

5 NAME OF THE PATIENT

6 ADDRESS OF THE PATIENT

7 AGE OF THE PATIENT if under 12 years old.

DIAGRAM 6: PRESCRIPTION REQUIREMENTS

NB: Indelible – Prescriptions need to be written in indelible ink, for example they may be computer generated or typed.

NB: Private prescriptions – The diagram above bears the image of an NHS prescription; however, the same requirements apply to private prescriptions.

NB: Carbon copies – It is permissible to issue carbon copies of NHS prescriptions as long as they are signed in ink.

See section 3.3.5 for EEA and Swiss prescription requirements.

ADVANCED ELECTRONIC SIGNATURE

An advanced electronic signature is a signature that is linked uniquely to the signatory, capable of identifying the signatory and created using means over which the signatory can maintain sole control (Regulation 219(5) Human Medicines Regulations 2012). The Royal Pharmaceutical Society is unable to confirm whether or not individual systems are able to issue advanced electronic signatures. Suitable assurances should be obtained from the system manufacturer and business indemnity providers.

ELECTRONIC PRESCRIPTIONS

Detailed information on existing electronic prescription systems is available from the following websites:

Health and Social Care Information Centre: *Electronic Prescription Service (EPS)* **(www.hscic.gov.uk)**

Pharmaceutical Services Negotiating Committee (PSNC): *Electronic Prescription Service (EPS)* **(www.psnc.org.uk)**

NHS Education for Scotland: *Electronic Transfer of Prescriptions (ETP) Implementation Pack to Support eAMS* **(www.nes.scot.nhs.uk)**

NHS England. *Electronic Repeat Dispensing Guidance.* 2015. **(www.england.nhs.uk)**

Dispensing a prescription in Welsh language

Medicines legislation describes the requirements which need to be on a legally valid prescription. Language is not specified. There is currently no law or act that specifies that prescriptions in Wales have to be bilingual.

If the pharmacist is not a Welsh speaker and can't understand the prescription, the RPS advice is to put patient safety first. The pharmacist is responsible for finding the best way to help the patient. If the pharmacist is presented with a prescription they do not fully understand, this might be through translation services or informal networks. Some local health boards choose LanguageLine.

In the interests of patient safety, the RPS Welsh Pharmacy Board recommends that medicines should be labelled in English primarily to ensure that if a patient is seen by a non-Welsh speaker these important instructions are understood.

FURTHER READING

RPS. *Use of the Welsh language in pharmacy.* **(www.rpharms.com/resources-AtoZ)**

Repeatable prescriptions

NB: Repeatable prescriptions are a different concept from repeat prescribing for regular items made under the NHS repeat dispensing scheme (in England and Wales), and also different to instalment prescribing for Controlled Drugs (see section 3.7.7).

Repeatable prescriptions are prescriptions against which medicines can be dispensed more than once. NHS prescriptions are not repeatable. Prescriptions for Schedule 2 and 3 Controlled Drugs are not repeatable; however, prescriptions for Schedule 4 and 5 are repeatable. In this context the term 'repeatable' means the instance where the prescriber adds an instruction to the main prescription for the prescribed item to be repeated. This does not refer to the prescription counterpart which is sometimes used as a patient repeat request to the prescriber.

Private prescriptions can be repeated as indicated by the prescriber (e.g. repeat × 3 would indicate that the prescription could be dispensed a total of four times), but if the number of repeats is not stated then they can only be repeated once (i.e. the prescription could be dispensed twice in total). The only exception to this is a prescription for an oral contraceptive, which can (if the number of repeats is not specified) be dispensed six times (i.e. repeated five times) within six months of the appropriate date (see Diagram 6).

For other repeatable prescriptions (including Schedule 5 Controlled Drugs), the first dispensing must be made within six months of the appropriate date (for Schedule 4 Controlled Drugs the first dispensing is only valid for 28 days after the appropriate date), following which there is no legal time limit for the remaining repeats. However, pharmacists should use professional judgement, taking into consideration clinical factors, to determine whether further repeat dispensing is appropriate.

The patient can choose to have subsequent supplies made from different pharmacies on their repeat prescription. Therefore to maintain an audit trail we advise the pharmacist at the time of supply to mark on the prescription the date, name and address of the pharmacy from where supply has been made.

Prisons provide NHS healthcare; however, FP10 forms are not used. Therefore the NHS repeat dispensing scheme cannot be used unless in the very unlikely event use of FP10 has been authorised by the Prison Trust.

Validity of owings on prescriptions

Medicines must be supplied within a certain period from the appropriate date (i.e. the date on which the prescription was signed by the prescriber or the date indicated as being the start date), therefore any owed medicines should be supplied within this validity period.

Table 2 summarises the validity of owings on NHS and private prescriptions (please note that this table does not cover repeatable prescriptions, NHS repeat dispensing prescriptions in England and Wales or Controlled Drug instalment prescriptions).

TABLE 2: VALIDITY OF OWINGS ON NHS AND PRIVATE PRESCRIPTIONS

MEDICINE	VALIDITY OF OWING
PRESCRIPTION-ONLY MEDICINES (POM) AND CONTROLLED DRUGS SCHEDULE 5	6 months from the appropriate date (see 'Date' in Diagram 6, section 3.3.1)
PHARMACY (P) MEDICINES AND GENERAL SALE MEDICINES (GSL)	6 months from the appropriate date (see 'Date' in Diagram 6, section 3.3.1)*
SCHEDULE 2, 3 AND 4 CONTROLLED DRUGS (CD)	28 days after the appropriate date (see 'Date' in Diagram 13, section 3.7.7)

* Please note this is a professional requirement.

Record keeping

Private prescriptions for a POM must be retained for two years from the date of the sale or supply or for repeatable prescriptions from the date of the last sale or supply. Private prescriptions for Schedule 2 and 3 Controlled Drugs must be submitted to the relevant NHS agency (for further information see section 3.7.7). Records must be made in the POM register (written or electronically), which should be retained for two years from the date of the last entry in the register. The record must include:

- **SUPPLY DATE** – the date on which the medicine was sold or supplied
- **PRESCRIPTION DATE** – the date on the prescription
- **MEDICINE DETAILS** – the name, quantity, formulation and strength of medicine supplied (where not apparent from the name)
- **PRESCRIBER DETAILS** – the name and address of the practitioner
- **PATIENT DETAILS** – the name and address of the patient.

The record should be made on the day the sale or supply takes place or if that is not practical, on the next day following.

Prescriptions for oral contraceptives are exempt from record keeping; as are prescriptions for Schedule 2 Controlled Drugs where a separate Controlled Drug register record has been made (see section 3.7.11).

Annex D1: Health Records Retention Schedule from the Department of Health guidance titled *Records Management: NHS Code of Practice Part 1 and Part 2* details a minimum retention period for each type of health record (**www.gov.uk/government/publications/records-management-nhs-code-of-practice**)

Incomplete prescriptions

Details of the medicinal product (such as name, strength, form, quantity and dose) are not legal requirements for prescriptions for POMs. Clearly, however, they are important for identifying which medicine to supply, how much to supply and at what dose. It is also important from a prescription pricing and remuneration perspective.

Information on endorsing incomplete prescriptions is available in the following documents:

England: Pharmaceutical Services Negotiating Committee (PSNC) *Alphabetical Guide to Prescription Endorsement for Pharmacy Contractors Quick Reference Guide* (**www.psnc.org.uk**)

Scotland: Community Pharmacy Scotland *Endorsing Guidance for electronic and paper prescriptions* (**www.communitypharmacyscotland.org.uk**)

Wales: Shared Services Partnership *Alphabetical Guide to Prescription Endorsement* (**www.primarycareservices.wales.nhs.uk/pharmacy-services**)

PRESCRIPTIONS FOR DISCHARGED PRISONERS – ENGLAND

FP10 prescriptions are not allowed for patients while they are in prison (unless authorised by Prison Trust). However, those who are about to be discharged from prison without the usual methods for ensuring continuity of supply of their medicines (e.g. those released unexpectedly from court, those who fail to obtain a take-out supply of their medicines or those who fail to obtain a same or next day prescribing appointment with a drug treatment agency) can be given an FP10 or FP10[MDA] prescription to take to their community pharmacy. These FP10 forms have the name and address of the prison printed on them and the patient is exempt from payment by virtue of having HMP in the address.

For more information, the Department of Health has produced guidance entitled *Provision of FP10 and FP10[MDA] prescription forms by HM Prison Service for released prisoners* (available under National Archives at **http://webarchive.nationalarchives.gov.uk/20130123193253/http://www.dh.gov.uk/en/Publicationsandstatistics/Publications/PublicationsPolicyAndGuidance/DH_083474**)

3.3.2 FAXED PRESCRIPTIONS

A 'fax' of a prescription does not fall within the definition of a legally valid prescription within human medicines legislation because it is not written in indelible ink and has not been signed in ink by an appropriate practitioner. Supplying medicines against a 'fax' is associated with considerable risks;

1. Uncertainty that the supply has been made in accordance with a legally valid prescription.

2. Risks of poor reproduction.

3. Risks of non-receipt of the original prescription and therefore inability to demonstrate that a supply had been made in accordance with a prescription.

4. Risks that the original prescription is subsequently amended by the prescriber in which case the supply would not have been made in accordance with the prescription.

5. Risks the 'fax' is sent to multiple pharmacies and duplicate supplies are made.

6. Risks that the prescription is not genuine.

7. Risks that the system of sending and receiving of the 'fax' is not secure.

Alternative mechanisms for the supply of medicines in an emergency exist for pharmacists working in registered pharmacies and can achieve a similar outcome in many scenarios with a better risk profile. Where this option can be used, it should be used.

Electronic prescriptions are also recognised in Human Medicines Regulations 2012 and where a system is being developed should be considered as an option.

Pharmacists considering supplying medicines against a fax should make an informed decision and take steps to safeguard patient safety, and where possible mitigate the risks identified above. Where appropriate, you should consider making a record of the decision-making process and your reasons leading to a particular course of action.

The supply of Schedule 2 and 3 Controlled Drugs without possession of a lawful prescription could be prosecuted as a criminal offence.

FURTHER RESOURCES

Further information on additional safeguards used in sectors such as 'secure environments' and secondary care may be available from specialist groups (see section 7) or from the specialist virtual networks on the RPS website (**www.rpharms.com**)

3.3.3 DENTAL PRESCRIPTIONS

Dentists can legally write prescriptions for any POM. However, the General Dental Council advises that dentists should restrict their prescribing to areas in which they are competent and generally only prescribe medicines that have uses in dentistry.

When prescribing on an NHS dental prescription, dentists are restricted to the medicines listed in the Dental Prescribers' Formulary (Part 8a of the Drug Tariff for Scotland or Part XVIIa of the Drug Tariff for England and Wales). The dental formulary is also reproduced within the British National Formulary.

3.3.4 FORGED PRESCRIPTIONS

Although it can be difficult to detect a forged prescription, every pharmacist should be alert to the possibility that any prescription could be a forgery.

The following checklist may be useful to help detect fraudulent prescriptions and prompt further investigation:

- Is a large or excessive quantity prescribed and is this appropriate for the medicine and condition being treated?
- Is the prescriber known?
- Is the patient known?
- Has the title 'Dr' been inserted before the signature?
- Is the behaviour of the patient indicative? (e.g. nervous, agitated, aggressive, etc)
- Is the medicine known to be commonly misused?

Further investigation may be necessary. The following are appropriate actions to take:

1. Scrutinise the signature carefully – possibly checking against a known genuine prescription from the same prescriber.
2. Confirm details with the prescriber (e.g. whether or not a prescription has been issued, the original intention of the prescriber and whether or not there has been an alteration).
3. Use contact details for the prescriber that are obtained from a source other than the suspicious prescription (e.g. directory enquiries).

Reporting concerns

Depending upon the nature of the fraudulent prescription, use your professional judgement to assess whether or not it is a matter that requires referral to the police, NHS Counter Fraud Services (for NHS prescriptions only) or whether the matter can be resolved by discussions with the patient and prescriber.

FURTHER READING

Further information on NHS Protect is available at (**www.nhsbsa.nhs.uk/protect.aspx**)

Further information on NHS Scotland Counter Fraud Services is available at (**www.cfs.scot.nhs.uk**)

Further information on NHS Counter Fraud Services Wales is available at (**www.wales.nhs. uk/sitesplus/955/page/63057**)

3.3.5 PRESCRIPTIONS FROM THE EEA OR SWITZERLAND

Prescriptions issued by a doctor, dentist, prescribing pharmacist* or prescribing nurse* registered in an EEA country (for a list of EEA countries see box) or Switzerland are legally recognised in the UK. Emergency supplies for

LIST OF EEA COUNTRIES

Austria, Belgium, Bulgaria, Croatia, Cyprus, Czech Republic, Denmark, Estonia, Finland, France, Germany, Greece, Hungary, Iceland, Ireland, Italy, Latvia, Liechtenstein, Lithuania, Luxembourg, Malta, Netherlands, Norway, Poland, Portugal, Romania, Slovakia, Slovenia, Spain, Sweden.

patients of the above healthcare professionals registered in an EEA country or Switzerland are also permitted. Prescriptions from the EEA or Switzerland can be repeatable, see section 3.3.1 for further information on repeatable prescriptions.

*Where they exist.

Prescription requirements

From 31 March 2014 the following details are required on a prescription from the healthcare professionals outlined above:

- **PATIENT DETAILS:** Patient's full first name(s), surname and date of birth

- **PRESCRIBER DETAILS:** Prescriber's full first name(s), surname, professional qualifications, direct contact details including email address and telephone or fax number (with international prefix), work address (including the country they work in)

- **PRESCRIBED MEDICINE(S) DETAILS:** Name of the medicine (brand name where appropriate), pharmaceutical form, quantity, strength and dosage details

- **PRESCRIBER SIGNATURE**

- **DATE OF ISSUE:** Vaild for up to six months from the appropriate date (prescriptions for Schedule 4 Controlled Drugs 28 days). For prescriptions from these countries the appropriate date is the date on which the prescription was signed.

Please note: Even if the prescription requirements have been written in a foreign language the prescription is still legally acceptable. However, the pharmacist needs to have enough information to enable the safe supply of medicines considering patient care and wellbeing.

Medicines not available on an EEA prescription

Schedule 1, 2 and 3 Controlled Drugs and medicinal products without a marketing authorisation valid in the UK, cannot be dispensed in the UK when prescribed by a doctor, dentist, prescribing pharmacist or prescribing nurse registered in an EEA country or Switzerland.

Consider referral to an appropriate UK-registered prescriber if such items are requested.

Checking the registration status of EEA or Swiss prescriber

A pan-EEA database of prescribers does not exist and, indeed, not all of the other EEA countries have a register of practitioners or online registers in English. Therefore, it may not always be possible to check the registration of an EEA or Swiss prescriber. However, up-to-date contact details for EEA competent authorities to check registration details of the following healthcare professionals can be obtained from:

- Doctors: General Medical Council (GMC) **www.gmc-uk.org** (search for 'EEA evidence of qualifications')
- Dentists: General Dental Council (GDC) **www.gdc-uk.org** (search for 'List of EEA competent authorities')
- Nurses: Nursing and Midwifery Council (NMC) **www.nmc.org.uk** (search for 'Trained in Europe').

Inability to confirm registration status

If it is not possible to confirm the registration status of the EEA prescriber after taking all reasonable steps to do so, then it may still be possible to make a safe and legal supply in the interests of patient care. It would be beneficial to keep a record of the details of any interventions and steps taken. This would require checking (and being satisfied) that prescription requirements are fulfilled, questioning the patient and careful use of professional judgement. A 'due diligence' defence exists for EEA prescriptions. However, only a court could decide, ultimately on a case-by-case basis, whether due diligence has been exercised.

Emergency supply

Emergency supplies at the request of a patient, or at the request of the EEA or Swiss prescriber, are legally possible.

The usual emergency supply process (see section 3.3.10.2) should be used and, where the request originates from an EEA prescriber, then a prescription needs to be received within 72 hours. Remember that Schedule 1, 2 and 3 (including phenobarbital) cannot be supplied to a patient. A Schedule 4 and 5 Controlled Drug can be supplied as an emergency supply to a patient of an EEA or Swiss prescriber.

Referral

It is important to bear in mind that the legislation outlined above is enabling – it is not obligatory to dispense an EEA or Swiss prescription if presented with one. If a pharmacist is not satisfied that a prescription is clinically appropriate, or legally valid, and an emergency supply is not appropriate, then a valid alternative remains to refer the patient to a prescriber based in the UK.

3.3.6 MILITARY PRESCRIPTIONS

Military primary healthcare medical centres are broadly similar to Dispensing Doctors practices in the NHS, where the doctor in charge delegates the dispensing function to a suitably trained individual. However, only large medical centres have retained their in-house dispensary. The remaining, smaller medical centres have outsourced the dispensing process to designated community pharmacies under a Ministry of Defence (MOD) contract. Community pharmacies not covered by the contract will not routinely handle military prescriptions.

Military prescriptions are written on a military form FMed 296, see Diagram 7.

Pharmacies with a dispensing contract with the MOD will usually invoice the MOD directly.

In the unusual event that an FMed 296 is presented to a non-contracted pharmacy, then the prescription should be treated as a private prescription. In these circumstances, non-contracted pharmacies are not to invoice the MOD directly but are to charge the patient the appropriate fee. It is then up to the individual patient to recover any costs incurred from their military unit (please note: this practice should only be used in exceptional circumstances). Similarly, any military personnel that presents an NHS or other private prescription (including using an FMed 296 as a private prescription) should pay the appropriate fee and request a receipt to reclaim any costs, if eligible. This is unless, of course, for an NHS prescription they fall into an NHS exemption category and present an exemption certificate.

All Controlled Drug prescriptions are written on designated standardised forms, which individual prescribers obtain from their local primary care organisations or NHS Health Boards in the same manner as all other prescribers wishing to prescribe CDs privately (see section 3.7.7).

If there is any doubt to the validity of the FMed 296, normal procedures should be employed (see section 3.3.4).

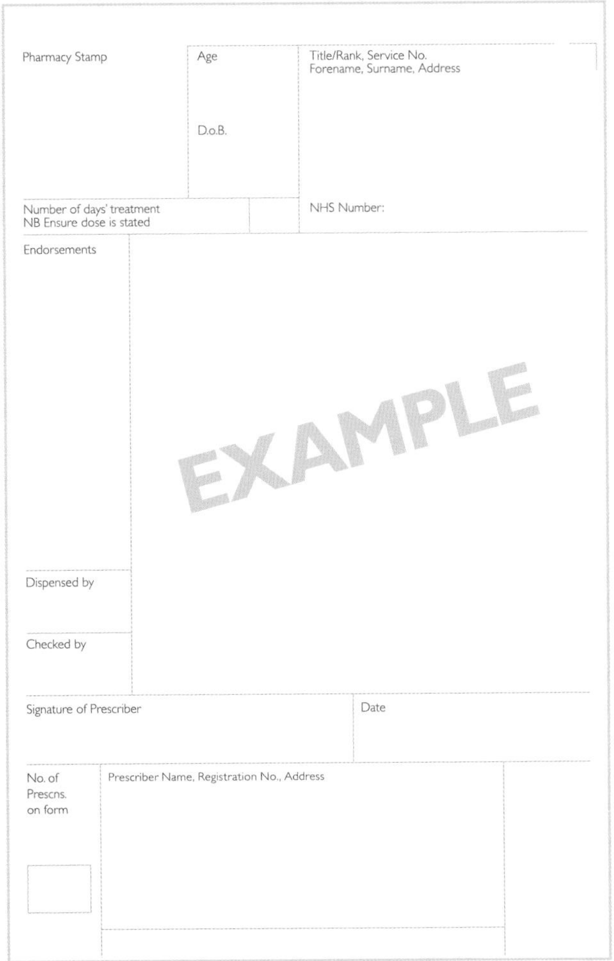
Pharmacy Stamp
Age
D.o.B.
Title/Rank, Service No.
Forename, Surname, Address
Number of days' treatment
NB Ensure dose is stated
NHS Number:
Endorsements
EXAMPLE
Dispensed by
Checked by
Signature of Prescriber
Date
No. of Prescns. on form
Prescriber Name, Registration No., Address

DIAGRAM 7: EXAMPLE OF AN FMED 296 PRESCRIPTION

Particular attention should be paid in the following circumstances:

- **Handwritten FMed 296.** The majority of FMed 296 prescriptions will be computer generated. It is highly unusual to see handwritten prescriptions, especially for MOD accountable drugs (these include Schedule 3, 4 and 5 Controlled Drugs, codeine, sedatives and medicines for erectile dysfunction)
- **British Forces Post Office (BFPO) address stamp.** Prescriptions with a BFPO address stamp have been generated abroad and are normally not seen in the UK. If there is any doubt, pharmacists are advised to check the registration status of the doctor, dentist or independent prescriber (see section 3.3.16).

When a medicinal product is dispensed there is a legal requirement for the following to appear on the dispensing label:

- Name of the patient
- Name and address of the supplying pharmacy
- Date of dispensing
- Name of the medicine
- Directions for use
- Precautions relating to the use of the medicine.
- The RPS recommends the following also appears on the dispensing label:
- 'Keep out of the sight and reach of children'
- 'Use this medicine only on your skin' where applicable.

NB: In secure environments it is strongly recommended that the prisoner number is also included on the label as a definitive patient identifier.

Additional information can be added to the dispensing label if the pharmacist considers it to be necessary.

OUTER CONTAINER Whilst it is lawful to label the outer container, we advise that the labelling recommendations of the National Patient Safety Agency are followed. These guidelines raise the issue that the outer container may be discarded and, therefore, the labelling information could be lost, so the actual container (e.g. inhaler or tube of cream) should be labelled rather than the outer container.

OPTIMISATION OF LABELLING Subject to the professional skill and judgement of a pharmacist, if he/she is of the opinion that the directions for use, name or common name of the medicine, or precautions, relating to the use of the medicine, are not appropriate on the prescription, they can substitute these with appropriate particulars of a similar kind when producing the dispensing label without contacting the prescriber.

It would be good practice to make a record to maintain a clinical audit trail underpinning patient care.

It is important to understand that the above is enabling and not mandatory. The options to contact the prescriber or refer the patient to the prescriber remain available and should be used where this is appropriate in the opinion of the pharmacist having exercised professional skill and judgement.

Full details can be viewed in '*Optimising Dispensing Labels and Medicines Use – quick reference guide. 2012*' on the RPS website at **www.rpharms.com/resources-AtoZ**.

Assembly and pre-packing medicines

The assembly or pre-packing of medicines by the pharmacy to be supplied to a separate legal entity (e.g. for a NHS Trust to supply a different NHS Trust or an out of hours medical practice) requires the appropriate licence from the MHRA (i.e. Manufacturer's/importer's licence (MIA) or Manufacturer 'specials' licence (MS)). The MHRA can be contacted for further details on the licence and any additional requirements (**www.gov.uk/government/organisations/medicines-and-healthcare-products-regulatory-agency**).

For activities that include over-labelling for supply, the RPS would also advise you contact the MHRA for further details.

Labelling of medicines broken down from bulk containers for dispensing

Pharmacists are able to break down bulk containers into smaller quantities more appropriate for dispensing against prescriptions which have already been received and are being dispensed or in anticipation of these prescriptions. For the latter case medicines must be labelled with the:

- Name of the medicine
- Quantity of the medicine in the container
- Quantitative particulars of the medicine (i.e. the ingredients)
- Handling and storage requirements where appropriate
- Expiry date
- Batch reference number (e.g. LOT number or BN).

The medicines which have been broken down from bulk need to be labelled with usual labelling requirements upon dispensing.

If both of the above (**Assembly and pre-packing medicines and Labelling of medicines broken down from bulk containers for dispensing**) do not apply to you, you should contact the MHRA for further information.

National Patient Safety Agency. *Design for patient safety: A guide to the design of dispensed medicines.* January 2007. **(www.npsa.nhs.uk)**

MHRA. *Best practice guidance on the labelling and packaging of medicines.* 2014. Available at **(www.gov.uk/government/ organisations/medicines-and-healthcare-products- regulatory-agency)**

MHRA. *Additional warning statements for inclusion on the label and/or in the leaflet of certain medicines.* 2014. **(www.gov.uk/government/organisations/ medicines-and-healthcare-products-regulatory- agency)**

National Patient Safety Agency. *Design for patient safety: a guide to the design of the dispensing environment.* January 2007. **(www.npsa.nhs.uk)**

NICE. *Medicines practice guidelines: Patient Group Directions.* August 2013. **(www.nice.org.uk)**

3.3.8 ADMINISTRATION

The Human Medicines Regulations 2012 prevents a person administering a parenteral POM to another person unless they are acting in accordance with the directions of an appropriate practitioner. However, there are exemptions to this restriction.

The legislation allows the administration of listed parenteral medicines to human beings in an emergency for the purpose of saving life. The list of medicines for use by parenteral administration in an emergency can be found in Schedule 19 of The Human Medicines Regulations 2012 **(www.legislation.gov.uk)**.

An example is administering adrenaline injection 1 in 1000 (1mg/ml) for the emergency treatment of anaphylaxis (see section 3.5.17 for further information).

Further exemptions apply to the administration of smallpox vaccine or administration linked to medical exposure (including radioactive medicines), and to specific classes of persons (such as midwives and paramedics) for specified parenteral POMs under certain conditions.

Medicines legislation does not restrict who can administer non-parenteral POMs (i.e. oral, inhaled, topical or rectal dosage forms, etc). However, in most healthcare settings, the person administering the medicine should only do so with the authority of a prescription, patient specific direction or patient group direction and should be appropriately trained.

The Human Medicines Regulations 2012 provides a range of exemptions to the restrictions on the sale, supply and administration of medicines.

A number of these exemptions are collectively described as patient specific directions (PSDs).

Legislation does not specifically define a PSD. However, it is generally accepted to mean a written instruction from a doctor, dentist or other independent prescriber for a medicine to be supplied or administered to a named patient after the prescriber has assessed that patient on an individual basis.

Some organisations may limit who is authorised to supply and/or administer medicines under a PSD within their local medicines policies and governance arrangements. Any trained and competent health professional would be suitable. PSDs relate to a specific named patient but do not need to comply with the requirements specified for a prescription.

In a hospital ward, written PSDs are encountered on inpatient charts as directions to administer. While the law does not stipulate what should be included in a PSD, sufficient information must be available for the person administering the specified medicine to do so safely. In addition a PSD, if sufficiently clear, may also be a direction to make a sale or supply.

Typically the directions within an inpatient chart are transcribed onto an order form for the pharmacy to prepare discharge ('take home') medicines. The pharmacist in this instance is not prescribing, and the supply is made under the authority of the original written direction to supply. Transcription should be carried out or counter-checked by a pharmacist. This order form does not replace a discharge letter; however, it can form part of the discharge letter.

For the purpose of administration (rather than supply) it is also possible for the directions of an appropriate practitioner to be verbal or telephoned. This is because medicines legislation does not specify that the authorisation to administer a medicine needs to be in writing. Nevertheless, a written authorisation should be used wherever possible and any applicable standards that require the authorisation to be in writing should be adhered to. For example, in England, the Care Quality Commission fundamental standards, and the standards of any relevant healthcare professionals involved in administration (e.g. nurses) will be applicable.

Some hospitals have formulated policies to permit, in an emergency, the administration of medicines following a telephoned or verbal request from an appropriate practitioner – usually involving two nurses checking one another.

Some hospitals have also formulated policies for the supply and/or administration of POMs (and P or general sale medicines) to ensure that medicines are handled safely, securely and appropriately. Such policies should be carefully considered and agreed by medical, nursing and pharmacy staff to ensure that patients are not put at risk. The policy should be cross-referenced against standards set by any applicable body, including regulatory and professional bodies of relevant healthcare professionals involved in the process. If in doubt, the Department of Health should be consulted for hospitals in England (along with the hospital's legal advisors). Hospitals in Scotland should contact the Scottish Executive, while hospitals in Wales should contact the Department of Health and Social Services.

British Medical Association. *Patient group directions and patient specific directions in general practice.* January 2016. **(www.bma.org.uk)**

Online resources are available on the NHS Education for Scotland website **(www.nes.scot.nhs.uk)**

Department of Health (National Archives). *Medicine matters: A guide to mechanisms for the prescribing, supply and administration of medicines.* July 2006. **(http://webarchive.nationalarchives. gov.uk/20130107105354/http:/www.dh.gov. uk/en/Publicationsandstatistics/Publications/ PublicationsPolicyAndGuidance/DH_064325)**

Online resources are available on the Care Quality Commission website **(www.cqc.org.uk)**

Nursing and Midwifery Council. *Standards for medicines management.* 2010. **(www.nmc.org.uk)**

3.3.10 EXEMPTIONS: SALE AND SUPPLY WITHOUT A PRESCRIPTION

3.3.10.1 PATIENT GROUP DIRECTIONS

3.3.10.2 EMERGENCY SUPPLY

3.3.10.3 PANDEMIC EXEMPTIONS

3.3.10.4 OPTOMETRIST OR PODIATRIST SIGNED ORDERS FOR PATIENTS

3.3.10.5 SUPPLY OF SALBUTAMOL INHALERS TO SCHOOLS

3.3.10.6 SUPPLY OF NALOXONE BY INDIVIDUALS PROVIDING RECOGNISED DRUG TREATMENT SERVICES

The preferred way for patients to receive medicines is for an appropriately qualified healthcare professional to prescribe for an individual patient on a one-to-one basis. There are, however, several exemptions that allow POMs to be sold or supplied without a prescription. Pharmacists are likely to be involved in many of these mechanisms and need to be aware of:

- Patient group directions (PGDs)
- Patient specific directions (see section 3.3.9)
- Emergency supplies
- Pandemic exemptions
- Optometrist or podiatrist signed orders for patients
- Supply of salbutamol inhalers to schools
- Supply of naloxone by individuals providing recognised drug treatment services.

3.3.10.1 Patient group directions

A PGD is a written direction that allows the supply and/or administration of a specified medicine or medicines, by named authorised health professionals, to a well-defined group of patients requiring treatment for a specific condition.

It is important that pharmacists involved with PGDs understand the scope and limitations of PGDs as well as the wider context into which they fit to ensure safe, effective services for patients.

The supply and administration of medicines under a PGD should only be reserved for those limited situations where this offers an advantage for patient care, without compromising patient safety.

A PGD should only be developed after careful consideration of all the potential methods of supply and/or administration of medicines, including prescribing, by medical or non-medical prescribers.

Since the 23 April 2012, pharmacists have been empowered by legislation to supply, offer to supply and administer diamorphine or morphine under a PGD for the immediate, necessary treatment of sick or injured persons. Further information about this is available from the NHS PGD website.

FURTHER READING

Online resources are available at the NHS PGD Website (**www.medicinesresources.nhs.uk/en/ Communities/NHS/PGDs/?id=512054**)

NICE. *Medicines practice guidelines: Patient Group Directions.* August 2013. (**www.nice.org.uk**)

National Prescribing Centre (UK Web Archive). *Patient group directions.* December 2009. (**http://www.webarchive.org.uk/wayback/ archive/20140627112220/http:/www.npc.nhs.uk/non_ medical/resources/patient_group_directions.pdf**)

NHS Education for Scotland. *Patient group directions.* (**http://www.nes.scot.nhs.uk/ education-and-training/by-theme-initiative/ prescribing-and-patient-group-direction/ patient-group-directions.aspx**)

MHRA. *Patient group directions: who can use them.* December 2014. (**www.gov.uk/government/ publications/patient-group-directions-pgds**)

MHRA (National Archives). *Advice on administering eye drops in retinal screening programmes.* 2012. (**http://webarchive. nationalarchives.gov.uk/20141205150130/http:// www.mhra.gov.uk/Howweregulate/Medicines/ Availabilityprescribingsellingandsupplyingofmedicines/ Frequentlyraisedissues/index.htm**)

3.3.10.2 Emergency supply

In an emergency and under certain conditions a pharmacist working in a registered pharmacy can supply POMs to a patient without a prescription if requested by a prescriber or the patient.

Pharmacists should consider each request on a case-by-case basis, using their professional judgement to decide which course of action they believe will be in the best interest of the patient.

In Scotland, a national PGD is in place that allows participating pharmacies and pharmacists to supply medicines for the urgent provision of current repeat medicines, appliances and ACBS (borderline) items (**www.communitypharmacy.scot.nhs.uk/unscheduled_ care.html**). Therefore, pharmacists working in Scotland are only likely to use the standard emergency supply exemptions (outlined below) for patients who are not eligible for treatment under the national PGD.

An equivalent national PGD in England and Wales has not been established.

EMERGENCY SUPPLY AT THE REQUEST OF A PRESCRIBER

Doctors, dentists, supplementary prescribers, community practitioner nurse prescribers, nurse independent prescribers, optometrist independent prescribers, pharmacist independent prescribers, physiotherapist independent prescribers, podiatrists independent prescribers, therapeutic radiographer independent prescribers and EEA or Swiss doctors, dentists, prescribing pharmacist and prescribing nurse can all authorise an emergency supply under certain conditions. The conditions are:

- **APPROPRIATE PRESCRIBER** – the pharmacist is satisfied that the request is from one of the prescribers stated above

- **EMERGENCY** – the pharmacist is satisfied that a prescription cannot be provided immediately due to an emergency (e.g. patient cannot collect the prescription from the prescriber, the prescriber is unable to drop off prescription at the pharmacy and patient urgently needs the medicine(s), etc.)

- **PRESCRIPTION WITHIN 72 HOURS** – the prescriber agrees to provide a written prescription within 72 hours

- **DIRECTIONS** – the medicine is supplied in accordance with the direction given by the prescriber

- **NOT FOR CONTROLLED DRUGS, EXCEPT PHENOBARBITAL** – Schedule 1, 2 or 3 Controlled Drugs cannot be supplied in an emergency with the exception of phenobarbital (also known as phenobarbitone or phenobarbitone sodium) for epilepsy by a UK-registered doctor, dentist, supplementary prescriber and independent pharmacist or nurse prescriber. EEA doctors, dentists, prescribing pharmacists and prescribing nurses cannot request an emergency supply for any Schedule 1, 2, or 3 Controlled Drugs (including phenobarbital for any purpose) or medicinal products without a marketing authorisation valid in the UK

- **RECORD KEPT** – an entry must be made into the POM register on the day of the supply (or, if impractical, on the following day). The entry needs to include:

- the date the POM was supplied

- the name (including strength and form where appropriate) and quantity of medicine supplied

- the name and address of the prescriber requesting the emergency supply

- the name and address of the patient for whom the POM was required

- the date on the prescription (this can be added to the entry when the prescription is received by the pharmacy)

- the date on which the prescription is received (this should be added to the entry when the prescription is received in the pharmacy)

- **LABELLING** – usual labelling requirements apply (see section 3.3.7).

EMERGENCY SUPPLY AT THE REQUEST OF A PATIENT

Emergency supplies are also possible at the request of a patient if they have previously been prescribed the medicine by one of the following types of prescriber: doctor, dentist, supplementary prescriber, community practitioner nurse prescriber, nurse independent prescriber, optometrist independent prescriber, pharmacist independent prescriber, physiotherapist independent prescribers, podiatrists independent prescribers and EEA or Swiss doctor, dentist, prescribing pharmacist or prescribing nurse.

The supply can be made in the following circumstances:

- **INTERVIEW** – Regulation 225 Human Medicines Regulations 2012 requires a pharmacist to interview the patient. The RPS recognises that in some circumstances this might not be possible, for example if the patient is a child, or being cared for, etc. In these circumstances the RPS advises pharmacists to use their professional judgement and consider the best interest of the patient

- **IMMEDIATE NEED** – the pharmacist must be satisfied that there is an immediate need for the POM and that it is not practical for the patient to obtain a prescription without undue delay

  Legislation does not prevent a pharmacist from making an emergency supply when a doctor's surgery is open. As with any request for an emergency supply, pharmacists must consider the best interests of the patient. Where a pharmacist believes that it would be impracticable in the circumstances for a patient to obtain a prescription without undue delay they may decide that an emergency supply is necessary. Automatically referring patients who are away from home and have forgotten or run out of their medication to the nearest local surgery to register as a temporary resident may not always be the most appropriate course of action.

- **PREVIOUS TREATMENT** – the POM requested must previously have been used as a treatment and prescribed by at least one of the types of prescribers listed above

  (NB: The time interval from when the medicine was last prescribed to when it is requested as an emergency supply would need to be considered and you should use your professional judgement to decide whether a supply or referral to a prescriber is appropriate)

- **DOSE** – the pharmacist must be satisfied of knowing the dose that the patient needs to take (e.g. refer to the PMR, electronic health record, prescription repeat slip, labelled medicine box, etc.)

- **NOT FOR CONTROLLED DRUGS, EXCEPT PHENOBARBITAL** – phenobarbital can be supplied to patients of UK-registered prescribers for the purpose of treating epilepsy. Medicinal products cannot be supplied if they consist of or contain any other Schedule 1, 2 or 3 Controlled Drugs or the substances listed below: ammonium bromide, calcium bromide, calcium bromidolactobionate, embutramide, fencamfamin hydrochloride, fluanisone, hexobarbitone, hexobarbitone sodium, hydrobromic acid, meclofenoxate hydrochloride, methohexitone sodium, pemoline, piracetam, potassium bromide, prolintane hydrochloride, sodium bromide, strychnine hydrochloride, tacrine hydrochloride, thiopentone sodium

  (NB: Requests made by a patient of an EEA or Swiss doctor, dentist, prescribing pharmacist or prescribing nurse cannot be supplied if they are for medicines that do not have a marketing authorisation valid in the UK – see section 3.3.5)

- **LENGTH OF TREATMENT** – if the emergency supply is for a Controlled Drug (i.e. phenobarbital or Schedule 4 or 5 Controlled Drug), the maximum quantity that can be supplied is for five days' treatment. For any other POM, no more than 30 days can be supplied except in the following circumstances:

  - if the POM is insulin, an ointment, a cream, or an inhaler for asthma (i.e. the packs cannot be broken), the smallest pack available in the pharmacy should be supplied

  - if the POM is an oral contraceptive, a full treatment cycle should be supplied

- if the POM is an antibiotic in liquid form for oral administration, the smallest quantity that will provide a full course of treatment should be supplied

  (NB: Pharmacists should also consider whether it is appropriate to supply less than the maximum quantity allowed in legislation. Professional judgement should be used to supply a reasonable quantity that is clinically appropriate and lasts until the patient is able to see a prescriber to obtain a further supply)

- **RECORDS KEPT** – an entry must be made in the POM register on the day of the supply (or, if impractical, on the following day). The entry needs to include:

  - the date the POM was supplied

  - the name (including strength and form where appropriate) and quantity of medicine supplied

  - the name and address of the patient for whom the POM was supplied

  - information on the nature of the emergency, such as why the patient needs the POM and why a prescription cannot be obtained, etc.

- **LABELLING** – in addition to standard labelling requirements, the words 'Emergency supply' need to be added to the dispensing label.

OTHER POINTS TO CONSIDER WHEN FACED WITH REQUESTS FOR AN EMERGENCY SUPPLY

Pharmacists should be mindful of patients abusing emergency supplies (for example, where a patient medication record shows that a patient has requested a medicine as an emergency supply on several occasions).

It is possible to make an emergency supply even during surgery opening hours; trying to obtain a prescription can sometimes cause undue delay in treatment and, potentially, harm to the patient. If patients are away from home and have run out of their medicines, referring them to the nearest surgery to register as a temporary patient may not always be appropriate. An emergency supply can be made provided the conditions above are met.

REFUSAL TO SUPPLY

If a pharmacist decides not to make an emergency supply after gathering and considering the information discussed in this guidance, the patient should be advised on how to obtain a prescription for the medicine or appropriate medical care. This could involve referral to a doctor, NHS walk-in centre or to an Accident and Emergency department.

3.3.10.3 Pandemic exemptions

Legislation is in place that relaxes emergency supply
requirements in the event of a pandemic or imminent
pandemic being declared by the Department of Health.
It means that pharmacists would not need to interview the
patient who requires a medicine through emergency supply.

Provisions are also in place to allow the supply of medicines
against a protocol from designated collection points when
a disease is pandemic or imminently pandemic and there
is a serious or potentially serious risk to human health.
This would require an announcement by the Department
of Health in England, the Scottish Government or the Welsh
Assembly. These collection points would not need to be
registered pharmacy premises and supplies would not need
to take place under the supervision of a pharmacist.

Further information is available in Regulations 226 and
247 of the Human Medicines Regulations 2012
(www.legislation.gov.uk).

3.3.10.4 Optometrist or podiatrist signed orders for patients

Optometrists and podiatrists cannot authorise supplies of
POMs by writing prescriptions unless they are additionally
qualified as independent or supplementary prescribers.

However, pharmacists working in a registered pharmacy
can supply certain POMs directly to patients in accordance
with a signed order from any registered optometrist
or podiatrist.

The medicine requested must be one which can be legally
sold or supplied by the optometrist or podiatrist rather
than one which they can only administer. (NB: You cannot
supply medicines directly to patients which are on the
list of medicines that can only be administered by the
optometrist or podiatrist) (see MHRA website for list).

Please note: Optometrists who have undertaken
additional training and are accredited by the GOC as
'additional supply optometrists' can issue signed orders
for an extended range of medicines.

The signed order is not a prescription; therefore the
usual prescription requirements would not be needed.
However, you should be satisfied the optometrist or the
podiatrist has provided sufficient advice to enable the
patient to use the medicine safely and effectively.

If the supply is made, the pharmacist should ensure
that the medicine is labelled accordingly as a dispensed
medicinal product (see section 3.3.7), a patient information
leaflet is supplied to the patient and an appropriate record
is made in the POM register.

Any additional information or advice that enables the
patient to use the medicine safely and effectively should
also be provided if it has not already been provided by
the optometrist or podiatrist.

Details on how to check the registration of the
optometrist or podiatrist can be found in section 3.3.16.

The Association of Optometrists (contact details can be found at **www.aop.org.uk**)

MHRA. *Rules for the sale, supply and administration of medicines for specific healthcare professionals.* 2014. (**https://www.gov.uk/ government/publications/rules-for-the-sale-supply-and-administration-of-medicines/ rules-for-the-sale-supply-and-administration-of-medicines-for-specific-healthcare-professionals**)

Human Medicines Regulations 2012. *Schedule 17 Exemptions which apply to optometrists and podiatrists.* (**www.legislation.gov.uk**)

RPS. *Medicines that optometrists can order – quick reference guide.* 2012. (**www.rpharms. com/resources-AtoZ**)

RPS. *Supply of medicines to podiatrists and their patients – quick reference guide.* 2016. (**www. rpharms.com/resources-AtoZ**)

3.3.10.5 Supply of salbutamol inhalers to schools

Legislation came into force on 1 October 2014 that enables schools to hold stocks of salbutamol inhalers. These can then be supplied in an emergency by persons trained to administer them to pupils who are known to require such medication in schools.

WHO CAN PROVIDE A SIGNED ORDER FOR SALBUTAMOL INHALERS FOR A SCHOOL?

A written order signed by the principal or head teacher at the school must be provided to enable a supply to be made to the school.

WHAT INFORMATION SHOULD BE INCLUDED IN THE SIGNED ORDER?

In line with legislation requirements;

"The order must be signed by the principal or head teacher at the school concerned and state

(i) the name of the school for which the medicinal product is required,

(ii) the purpose for which that product is required, and

(iii) the total quantity required"

Ideally, appropriately headed paper should be used, however, this is not a legislative requirement.

HOW MANY INHALERS CAN A SCHOOL OBTAIN?

The number of inhalers that can be obtained by individual schools is not specified in legislation. As part of the consultation process it was acknowledged that the number held for emergency used would be dependent on a variety of factors including; the school size and the number of sites it is comprised of, the number of children known to have asthma, and past experiences of children who had not been able to access their inhaler. It was however agreed, generally that only a small number of inhalers were likely to be needed annually. Schools can purchase salbutamol inhalers from pharmacies provided it is for small quantities, on an occasional basis and not for profit thus in line with MHRA Guidance for pharmacists on the repeal of Section 10(7) of the Medicines Act 1968 (see also section 3.4).

WHAT RECORDS NEED TO BE KEPT IN THE PHARMACY?

The signed order needs to be retained for 2 years from the date of supply or an entry made into the Prescription-only-medicine (POM) register. Even where the signed order is retained it is good practice to make a record in the POM register for audit purposes. In line with normal record keeping requirements an entry in the POM register must include:

- Date the POM was supplied
- Name, quantity and where it is not apparent, formulation and strength of POM supplied
- Name and address, trade, business or profession of the person to whom the medicine was supplied
- The purpose for which it was sold or supplied.

WHAT OTHER INFORMATION COULD I BE ASKED TO PROVIDE?

The pharmacist could be also be asked to:

- Explain how to use a salbutamol inhaler and any associated information
- Advise schools on the selection of the most appropriate spacer device for the different age groups and how to use them correctly.

WHAT GUIDANCE IS AVAILABLE FOR SCHOOLS ON THE CHANGES?

The Department of Health has issued guidance outlining the principles of safe use of inhalers to capture the good practice which schools in England should observe **(https://www.gov.uk/government/publications/emergency-asthma-inhalers-for-use-in-schools)** and the Welsh Government has issued guidance that schools in Wales should observe **(http://learning.gov.wales/resources/browse-all/use-of-emergency-salbutamol-inhalers-in-schools-in-wales/?lang=en).** The guidance covers issues such as arrangements for storage, care and disposal of medication within the school environment. Although these guidance documents are mainly specific for England and Wales the principles of safe usage are however universal.

Schools in Scotland should contact their own regulator Education Scotland for further guidance on this where required **(http://www.educationscotland.gov.uk/).**

WHERE CAN I LOCATE INFORMATION ON A SCHOOL INCLUDING HEAD TEACHER/PRINCIPAL DETAILS IF REQUIRED?

There is no centralised database containing details of schools and head teachers across Great Britain. Possible sources of information would include:

- Department for Education's register of educational establishments in England and Wales **(www.education.gov.uk/edubase/home.xhtml)**
- Local authorities' directory of schools **(www.local.direct.gov.uk/LDGRedirect/Start.do?mode=1ols)**
- Ofsted reports **(www.reports.ofsted.gov.uk/)**
- Information on the individual school's website.

FURTHER INFORMATION

Asthma UK. (www.asthma.org.uk/)

NHS Choices. *Asthma in children.* (www.nhs.uk/Conditions/Asthma/)

Department for Education. *Supporting pupils at school with medical conditions. Statutory guidance for governing bodies of maintained schools and proprietors of academies in England.* 2014. (https://www.gov.uk/government/publications/supporting-pupils-at-school-with-medical-conditions--3)

Welsh Assembly. *Government Circular Access to Education and Support for Children and Young People with Medical Needs.* 2010. (http://gov.wales/topics/educationandskills/publications/guidance/medicalneeds/)

Scottish Executive. *The Administration of Medicines in Schools.* 2001. (http://www.gov.scot/Publications/)

RPS. *Supporting patients with Asthma – quick reference guide.* (www.rpharms.com/resources-AtoZ)

3.3.10.6 Supply of naloxone by individuals employed or engaged in the provision of recognised drug treatment services

Legislation came into force on 1 October 2015 that enables lawful drug treatment services to obtain naloxone from a wholesaler and people engaged or employed in their services to be able, as part of their role, to make a supply of naloxone available to patients for the purpose of it being available to save life in emergency, without a prescription, patient group direction (PGD) or patient specific direction (PSD).

For example, a worker in a lawful drug treatment service can supply naloxone for use in an emergency, to a family member or friend of a person using heroin, or to an outreach worker for a homelessness service whose clients include people who use heroin, without a prescription, PGD or PSD.

FURTHER INFORMATION

Department of Health, MHRA and Public Health England. *Widening the availability of naloxone.* November 2015. **(https://www. gov.uk/government/publications/widening- the-availability-of-naloxone/widening-the- availability-of-naloxone)**. This provides further information, including details of the services that are specified as lawful drug treatment services.

3.3.11 SELF-PRESCRIBED PRESCRIPTIONS AND PRESCRIPTIONS FOR CLOSE FRIENDS AND FAMILY

Pharmacists are occasionally requested to dispense medicines that have been self-prescribed by a prescriber or have been prescribed for close family and friends of the prescriber.

Although a prescription (including one for Controlled Drugs) in these circumstances may fulfil the usual legal requirements, pharmacists should consider the following before making a supply:

- It is generally considered poor practice to self-prescribe or to prescribe for persons for whom there is a close personal relationship

- The professional judgement of the prescriber may be impaired or influenced by the person they are prescribing for

- It may not be possible for a prescriber to conduct a proper clinical assessment on themselves or on close friends or family

- The regulatory body for doctors (General Medical Council) advises within the *Good Medical Practice* that doctors must wherever possible avoid prescribing for themselves or anyone with whom they have a close personal relationship

- The regulatory body for nurses (Nursing and Midwifery Council) advises within the document *Standards of proficiency for nurse and midwife prescribers* that nurses and midwives must not prescribe for themselves and, other than in exceptional circumstances, should not prescribe for anyone with whom they have a close personal or emotional relationship.

- Pharmacist prescribers should be aware of the following documents:

  - Department of Health *Improving Patients' Access to Medicines: A Guide to Implementing Nurse and Pharmacist Independent Prescribing within the NHS in England* (April 2006) states *'Pharmacist Independent Prescribers must not prescribe any medicine for themselves. Neither should they prescribe a medicine for anyone with whom they have a close personal or emotional relationship, other than in an exceptional circumstance'*

  - NHS Education for Scotland *A guide to good prescribing practice for prescribing pharmacists in NHS Scotland* (July 2012) states *'You must not prescribe for yourself or for anyone with whom you have a close personal or emotional relationship'*

- The existence and content of any local trust, board or hospital policy covering self-prescribing

- The abuse potential of the drug being requested

- Controlled drugs should only be supplied in exceptional circumstances and details documented. Where appropriate, the supply or request may prompt referral to the local Controlled Drug accountable officer.

In an emergency, after exercising professional judgement, a pharmacist may decide that it is appropriate to dispense a medicine that has been self-prescribed or prescribed for persons with whom the prescriber has a close personal relationship.

In the circumstance that refusing to supply is the most appropriate action, be prepared for the person requesting the supply to be disappointed. One strategy would be to clearly and calmly explain that in your professional judgement it would not be appropriate to supply the medicine.

In some circumstances where there is a risk of harm to patients or the public, there may be a duty to raise concerns to the appropriate body (e.g. General Medical Council) (see Appendix 6 for GPhC guidance on raising concerns).

FURTHER READING

Nursing and Midwifery Council. *Standards of proficiency for nurse and midwife prescribers.* April 2006. **(www.nmc.org.uk)**

Department of Health (National Archives). *Improving Patients' Access to Medicines: A Guide to Implementing Nurse and Pharmacist Independent Prescribing within the NHS in England.* (April 2006). **(http://webarchive.nationalarchives. gov.uk/20130107105354/http:/www.dh.gov. uk/en/Publicationsandstatistics/Publications/ PublicationsPolicyAndGuidance/DH_4133743)**

NHS Education for Scotland. *A guide to good prescribing practice for prescribing pharmacists in NHS Scotland.* (July 2012). **(www.nes. scot.nhs.uk/media/1457463/nesd0061_ goodprescribingpractice.pdf)**

General Medical Council. *Good medical practice.* 2013. **(www.gmc-uk.org)**

General Medical Council. *Good practice in prescribing and managing medicines and devices.* 2013. **(www.gmc-uk.org)**

Isotretinoin is a retinoid: when used orally to treat severe acne it has a high risk of causing severe and serious malformation of a foetus and also increases the risk of spontaneous abortion.

Pharmacists are involved in the dispensing of isotretinoin and in ensuring it is not used by women who might be pregnant or are considering becoming pregnant. A Pregnancy Prevention Programme (PPP) is in place to protect female patients at risk of pregnancy from becoming pregnant whilst using oral isotretinoin, and for at least one month after stopping oral isotretinoin.

The programme is a combination of education for healthcare professionals and patients, therapy management (including pregnancy testing before during and after treatment, contraception requirements) and distribution control.

Therapy should only be initiated by or under the supervision of a consultant dermatologist and under the conditions of the PPP. The prescriber must check that the patient complies with, understands and acknowledges the reasons for pregnancy prevention and agrees to monthly follow-up, contraceptive precautions and pregnancy testing.

Female patients should comply with the PPP conditions unless the prescriber agrees that there are compelling reasons that indicate there is no risk of pregnancy.

Reasons may include persons who cannot become pregnant, e.g. following a hysterectomy or a female who is not sexually active (and there is certainty that sexual activity will not start during the period of teratogenic risk).

SPECIAL DISTRIBUTION CONTROLS FOR FEMALES AT RISK OF PREGNANCY

1. **PRESCRIPTION VALIDITY** – under the PPP, prescriptions are valid only for seven days and ideally should be dispensed on the date the prescription is written. Prescriptions which are presented after seven days should be considered expired and the patient should be referred back to the prescriber for a new prescription. Pregnancy status may need to be reconfirmed by a further negative pregnancy test.

2. **QUANTITY** – check that the quantity is for a maximum of 30 days' supply. A quantity for more than 30 days can only be dispensed if the patient is confirmed by the prescriber as not being under the Pregnancy Prevention Programme.

In accordance with MHRA approved guidance, pharmacists should not accept repeat prescriptions, free sample distribution, or faxed prescriptions for oral isotretinoin. A telephone request should only be accepted if this is an emergency supply at the request of a PPP specialist prescriber together with confirmation that pregnancy status has been established as negative within the preceding seven days.

FURTHER RESOURCES

Full details of isotretinoin pregnancy prevention programmes are available on the 'Summary of Product Characteristics' for the oral isotretinoin preparation. Available at **(www.medicines.org.uk)**

British National Formulary **(wwwmedicinescomplete.com** or **www.evidence.nhs.uk)**

MHRA. Online oral retinoids (including isotretinoin) and pregnancy prevention resources for doctors, pharmacists and patients **(www.gov.uk/government/organisations/medicines-and-healthcare-products-regulatory-agency)**

RPS. *Dispensing oral isotretinoin and pregnancy prevention.* 2012. **(www.rpharms.com/resources-AtoZ)**

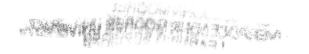

The Medicines and Healthcare Products Regulatory Agency (MHRA) issued a Drug Safety Update on 22 January 2015 *Medicines related to valproate: risk of abnormal pregnancy outcomes*. Pharmacists should familiarise themselves with this information on the risk of developmental disorders in children born to mothers who take sodium valproate during pregnancy and strengthened warnings relating to the use of valproate (sodium valproate, valproic acid and semi-sodium valproate) medicines.

To ensure female patients are aware of these risks, the MHRA have produced a toolkit. The toolkit includes a credit card sized patient card, a booklet for healthcare professionals, a checklist for prescribers and patients and a patient information booklet which advises patients to speak to their doctor or pharmacist if they have any questions.

Patients may approach their pharmacist for advice on the use of valproate medicines and when dispensing these, pharmacists should check whether female patients have had a discussion with their doctor about the new information relating to valproate medicines.

This guidance provides information on the advice that should be provided to safeguard all girls and women who use valproate. It does not cover the full list of contra-indications or full details of the risk information which can be found in the Summary of Product Characteristics of individual products and in the MHRA booklet for healthcare professionals (see *further reading*).

ADVICE FOR FEMALES

- Pharmacists should issue patients with the new credit card sized patient card (unless the patient already has one), and this can be used as an aid (together with other resources in the toolkit) to support discussions with patients. To reinforce her understanding you should encourage her to read the card and enter her details onto this. Manufacturers will distribute the alert cards to pharmacies

- Women of child-bearing age who are using valproate medicines should be advised on the use of effective contraception

- Those planning pregnancy should be advised to schedule an appointment with their prescriber to review treatment and to continue with contraception and valproate treatment in the meantime

- If there is an unplanned pregnancy whilst a patient is taking valproate medicines advise the patient NOT to stop their treatment and to arrange to see their prescriber urgently to review treatment

- Patients should be advised that treatment with valproate medicines should be reviewed regularly.

ADVICE FOR ALL PATIENTS (MALE AND FEMALE)

- Advise patient of the need for regular reviews and monitoring including liver function and full blood count. See the latest version of the BNF for further guidance

- Advise patients or their carers how to recognise the signs and symptoms of blood or liver disorders and pancreatitis, and to seek medical attention if these develop

- Remind patient to avoid abrupt withdrawal. Do not stop treatment without consulting their doctor – risk of status epilepticus and sudden unexpected death in epilepsy

- Patients should be advised that it is not recommended to drink alcohol whilst they are taking valproate medicines

- Pharmacists should provide driving advice for patients using valproate – see Patient Information Leaflet, Summary of Product Characteristics and DVLA pages listed under *further reading*.

ADDITIONAL CONSIDERATIONS

- Pharmacists are advised to report any suspected side effects to valproate medicines via the Yellow Card Scheme (see section 3.5.9 *Reporting adverse events*)

- The product literature and packaging for valproate medicines will be updated and pharmacists are reminded to ensure that patients have access to a Patient Information Leaflet. If pharmacists are supplying valproate medicines without the updated warnings on the packaging, they are advised to make patients or their carers aware of this, for example through use of the patient card

- Brand continuity in antiepileptic use: Consider the MHRA guidance *Antiepileptic drugs: changing between different manufacturers' products*

- People using services such as prescription collection and delivery are more likely to have little, if any, personal contact with the pharmacist. The RPS *Repeat medication management, prescription collection and delivery services* guidance provides advice on what to do in these scenarios **(www.rpharms.com/resources-AtoZ)**.

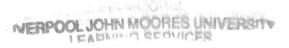

MHRA. Drug Safety Update. *Valproate and risk of abnormal pregnancy outcomes: new communication materials.* This includes links to the booklet for healthcare professionals, consultation checklist and card and guide to give to patients. **(https://www. gov.uk/drug-safety-update)**

MHRA Drug Safety Update. *Medicines related to valproate: risk of abnormal pregnancy outcomes.* January 2015. **(www.gov.uk/drug-safety-update)**

MHRA Drug Safety Update. *Antiepileptic drugs: new advice on switching between different manufacturers' products of a particular drug.* November 2013.
(www.gov.uk/drug-safety-update)

NICE Pathways. *Special considerations for girls and women with epilepsy.* 2015. **(http://pathways.nice.org.uk/)**

RPS and CPPE. *Medicines optimisation briefing – epilepsy.* January 2015. **(www.rpharms.com).**

Driver and Vehicle Licensing Agency. *DVLA'S Current medical guidelines: DVLA guidance for professionals* - see *bipolar disorder, epilepsy, neurological* and *psychiatric* appendices.
(www.gov.uk)

RPS. *New drugs and driving legislation: Advice for pharmacists and their patients.* 2015.
(www.rpharms.com/resources-AtoZ)
(see section 3.5.19 *Drugs and driving*).

electronic Medicines Compendium.
Summary of Product Characteristics and *Patient Information Leaflets* for individual products.
(www.medicines.org.uk/emc/).

3.3.14 EXPLAINING BIOSIMILAR MEDICINES

Recent advances in biotechnology have resulted in an increasing number of biological molecules and materials being used as medicines. This is a trend that is expected to continue, at least for the foreseeable future. A number of patents and periods of marketing exclusivity for biological medicines are expiring and biosimilar versions of the medicines are becoming more widely available e.g. insulin glargine. The introduction of biosimilars offers potential benefits in terms of cost savings for the NHS and increased access to treatments for patients. Biosimilars are not the same as a generic medicine and as a pharmacist you will need to be aware of the guidance around the use of biosimilars in order to ensure their safe and effective use.

WHAT IS A BIOLOGIC?

A biologic is a medicine made from a variety of natural sources that may be human, animal or microorganism in origin. Examples of a biologic include vaccines, blood and blood products, somatic cells, DNA, human cells and tissues and therapeutic proteins. In general, the first or original biologic on the market is termed the originator or reference product.

WHAT IS A BIOSIMILAR?

A biosimilar is a biologic medicine that is similar to an already licensed biologic medicine in terms of quality, safety and efficacy. A biosimilar is specifically developed and licensed to treat the same disease(s) as the original innovator product. A biosimilar can only be marketed after the patent protecting the originator product and any period of marketing exclusivity have expired.

WHY IS A BIOSIMILAR MEDICINE NOT A GENERIC MEDICINE?

Due to the complexity of structure and greater size of biologics as well as their inherent heterogeneity resulting from their production methods, it is not possible to make an identical copy of the originator biologic. Biosimilars are licensed for use based on extensive data on quality, safety and efficacy compared to the originator product. It is not possible to characterise a biologic to the same extent as a small molecule drug, where an identical copy can be produced, known as a generic medicine.

MEDICINES, ETHICS AND PRACTICE

IS IT POSSIBLE TO SWITCH BETWEEN AN ORIGINATOR BIOLOGIC AND A BIOSIMILAR?

Any decision to change the brand of a biologic used to treat a patient must only be made by a prescriber following discussions with the patient. It is recommended that, at the point of dispensing, the pharmacist confirms the patient has received the biologic they expect and that they are aware of how to store and use the medicine.

HOW WILL A BIOSIMILAR BE PRESCRIBED?

In contrast to generic products, all biosimilars will have their own unique brand name. The MHRA has recommended that all biologics should be prescribed by brand to avoid automatic substitution.

HOW ARE ADVERSE DRUG REACTIONS TO BIOSIMILARS REPORTED?

It is important that both the brand name and batch number of a biologic medicine are provided when reporting suspected adverse drug reactions to biologics to facilitate effective safety monitoring. To support patient safety, pharmacists should consider it good practice to record the brand name and batch number of any biologic medicine (including biosimilars) supplied to a patient.

TABLE 3: TABLE SHOWING EXAMPLES OF BIOLOGICS AND BIOSIMILARS

BIOLOGICS		
NON-PROPRIETARY NAME	ORIGINATOR PRODUCT	EXAMPLE OF BIOSIMILAR
insulin glargine	Lantus	Abasaglar
infliximab	Remicade	Inflectra/Remsima
filgrastim	Neupogen	Nivestim/Tevagrastim
epoetin alfa	Eprex	Binocrit/Retacrit
somatropin	Genotropin	Omnitrope

FURTHER INFORMATION

Diagrams illustrating the size and complexity of biosimilar medicines and a webinar on this subject can be found in **RPS**. *Explaining biosimilar medicines – quick reference guide*. 2015. (**www.rpharms.com/resources-AtoZ**)

British National Formulary (**www.medicinescomplete.com** or **www.evidence.nhs.uk**)

European Medicine Agency. *Questions and answers on biosimilar medicines (similar biological medicinal products)*. 2012. (**www.ema.europa.eu/ema**)

Association of the British Pharmaceutical Industry. *ABPI position on biological medicines, including biosimilar medicines*. 2015. (**www.abpi.org.uk**)

NICE. *Evaluation of biosimilar medicines*. 2015. (**www.nice.org.uk**)

NHS England. *What is a biosimilar medicine?* 2015. (**www.england.nhs.uk**)

British Generic Manufacturers Association. *Briefing paper on biosimilar medicines*. 2015. (**www.britishgenerics.co.uk**)

European Commission. *What you need to know about biosimilar medicinal products – a consensus information document*. 2013. (**http://ec.europa.eu**)

Healthcare Improvement Scotland and NHS Scotland. *Biosimilar medicines: A national prescribing framework*. 2015. (**www.healthcareimprovementscotland.org**)

MHRA Drug Safety Update. *High strength, fixed combination and biosimilar insulin products: minimising the risk of medication error*. 2015. (**www.gov.uk/drug-safety-update**)

TABLE 4: THE DIFFERENT TYPES OF PRESCRIBER AND RESTRICTIONS ON WHAT CAN BE PRESCRIBED

(All columns subject to considerations in other columns)

TYPE OF PRESCRIBER	CAN PRESCRIBE CONTROLLED DRUGS *(SCHEDULE 2 TO 5)* ON A PRESCRIPTION	CAN PRESCRIBE UNLICENSED MEDICINES	OTHER APPLICABLE CONSIDERATIONS	CAN AUTHORISE AN EMERGENCY SUPPLY FOR ITEMS WHICH CAN BE PRESCRIBED
DOCTOR REGISTERED IN THE UK	Yes. A Home Office licence is required to prescribe cocaine, dipipanone, or diamorphine for treating addiction Address of prescriber must be within the UK unless prescribing Schedule 4 or 5 Controlled Drugs	Yes (subject to accepted clinical good practice)	Clinical expertise	Yes. Includes phenobarbital for epilepsy but not Schedule 1, 2 and 3 Controlled Drugs (see section 3.3.10.2)
PHARMACIST INDEPENDENT PRESCRIBER	Yes (but not cocaine, dipipanone or diamorphine for treating addiction) Address of prescriber must be within the UK unless prescribing Schedule 4 or 5 Controlled Drugs	Yes (subject to accepted clinical good practice)	Medicines for any medical condition within their competence	Yes. Includes phenobarbital for epilepsy but not Schedule 1, 2 and 3 Controlled Drugs (see section 3.3.10.2)

TYPE OF PRESCRIBER	CAN PRESCRIBE CONTROLLED DRUGS (SCHEDULE 2 TO 5) ON A PRESCRIPTION	CAN PRESCRIBE UNLICENSED MEDICINES	OTHER APPLICABLE CONSIDERATIONS	CAN AUTHORISE AN EMERGENCY SUPPLY FOR ITEMS WHICH CAN BE PRESCRIBED
PHYSIOTHERAPIST INDEPENDENT PRESCRIBER	Only the following Controlled Drugs: diazepam, dihydrocodeine, lorazepam, oxycodone and temazepam for oral administration only; morphine for oral administration or for injection; fentanyl for transdermal administration	Only 'off-label' medicines subject to accepted clinical good practice	Medicines for any medical condition within their competence	Yes, but not Schedule 1, 2, and 3 Controlled Drugs, including phenobarbital (see section 3.3.10.2)
PODIATRISTS INDEPENDENT PRESCRIBER	Only the following Controlled Drugs for oral administration: diazepam, dihydrocodeine, lorazepam and temazepam	Only 'off-label' medicines subject to accepted clinical good practice	Medicines for any medical condition within their competence	Yes, but not Schedule 1, 2, and 3 Controlled Drugs, including phenobarbital (see section 3.3.10.2)
DENTIST REGISTERED IN THE UK	Yes (but not cocaine, dipipanone or diamorphine for treating addiction) Address of prescriber must be within the UK unless prescribing Schedule 4 or 5 Controlled Drugs	Yes (subject to accepted clinical good practice)	Should restrict prescribing to treatment of dental conditions but legally can prescribe within clinical expertise. NHS dental prescriptions are restricted to medicines within the Dental Formulary (See BNF)	Yes. Includes phenobarbital for epilepsy but not Schedule 1, 2 and 3 Controlled Drugs (see section 3.3.10.2)

TYPE OF PRESCRIBER	CAN PRESCRIBE CONTROLLED DRUGS *(SCHEDULE 2 TO 5)* ON A PRESCRIPTION	CAN PRESCRIBE UNLICENSED MEDICINES	OTHER APPLICABLE CONSIDERATIONS	CAN AUTHORISE AN EMERGENCY SUPPLY FOR ITEMS WHICH CAN BE PRESCRIBED
SUPPLEMENTARY PRESCRIBER (PHARMACIST, MIDWIFE, NURSE, CHIROPODIST, DIETITIAN, PODIATRIST, PHYSIOTHERAPIST, RADIOGRAPHER OR OPTOMETRIST)	Yes (but not cocaine, dipipanone or diamorphine for treating addiction) Address of prescriber must be within the UK unless prescribing Schedule 4 or 5 Controlled Drugs	Yes (subject to accepted clinical good practice)	Prescribed items are subject to clinical competence and inclusion within a clinical management plan agreed	Yes. Includes phenobarbital for epilepsy but not Schedule 1, 2 and 3 Controlled Drugs (see section 3.3.10.2)
NURSE INDEPENDENT PRESCRIBER	Yes (but not cocaine, dipipanone or diamorphine for treating addiction) Address of prescriber must be within the UK unless prescribing Schedule 4 or 5 Controlled Drugs	Yes (subject to accepted clinical good practice)	Medicines for any medical condition within their competence	Yes. Includes phenobarbital for epilepsy but not Schedule 1, 2 and 3 Controlled Drugs (see section 3.3.10.2)
OPTOMETRIST INDEPENDENT PRESCRIBER	No	Only 'off-label' medicines subject to accepted clinical good practice	For ocular conditions affecting the eye and surrounding tissue only	Yes
THERAPEUTIC RADIOGRAPHER INDEPENDENT PRESCRIBER	At the time of writing proposed changes to legislation in relation to the use of certain Controlled Drugs were still to be considered by the Home Office.	Only 'off label' medicines subject to accepted clinical good practice	Medicines for any medical condition within their competence	Yes, but not Schedule 1, 2 and 3 Controlled Drugs, including phenobarbital (see section 3.3.10.2)

TYPE OF PRESCRIBER	CAN PRESCRIBE CONTROLLED DRUGS *(SCHEDULE 2 TO 5)* ON A PRESCRIPTION	CAN PRESCRIBE UNLICENSED MEDICINES	OTHER APPLICABLE CONSIDERATIONS	CAN AUTHORISE AN EMERGENCY SUPPLY FOR ITEMS WHICH CAN BE PRESCRIBED
VETERINARY SURGEON AND VETERINARY PRACTITIONER	Yes (for the treatment of animals) Address of prescriber must be within the UK unless prescribing Schedule 4 or 5 Controlled Drugs Prescriptions for Schedule 2 and 3 Controlled Drugs must include the Royal College of Veterinary Surgeons registration number of the prescriber	Yes (for the treatment of animals – subject to the veterinary Cascade, see section 3.6)	For the treatment of animals only	Not applicable
EEA OR SWISS DOCTOR OR DENTIST	Schedule 4 and 5 Controlled Drugs only	No	Can only prescribe items which have a recognised marketing authorisation within the UK	Yes
COMMUNITY PRACTITIONER NURSE	No	No	Restricted to dressings, appliances and licensed medicines which are listed in the Nurse Prescribers' Formulary (see BNF)	Yes

NB: Schedule 1 Controlled Drugs can only be prescribed under Home Office licence.

3.3.16 CHECKING REGISTRATION OF HEALTHCARE PROFESSIONALS AND ADDITIONAL INFORMATION ON CONDITIONS OF SUPPLY

Pharmacists may need to verify the registration status of other pharmacists and other healthcare professionals as part of the due diligence process when checking whether a person can prescribe or whether they can be wholesaled to. Table 5 provides details on where registration information can be verified (along with additional relevant notes) for several types of healthcare professional.

TABLE 5: HOW TO CHECK REGISTRATION FOR HEALTHCARE PROFESSIONALS

HEALTHCARE PROFESSIONAL	WHERE TO CHECK REGISTRATION	COMMON ISSUES
PHARMACISTS	General Pharmaceutical Council **(www.pharmacyregulation.org)** 020 3713 8000	There are pharmacists with further qualifications, such as independent or supplementary prescribers, and this is reflected in the register
		Supplementary prescribers can prescribe all medicines included in a clinical management plan agreed with a prescriber and the patient. This includes Controlled Drugs and unlicensed medicines
		Independent prescribers can prescribe unlicensed medicines and since 23 April 2012 have also been able to prescribe Controlled Drugs. Prescribing should be restricted to areas of clinical competence
		Further information on non-medical prescribing, including FAQs, guidance and clinical management plans is available on the Department of Health website (National Archives) **(http://webarchive.nationalarchives.gov. uk/+/www.dh.gov.uk/en/Healthcare/ Medicinespharmacyandindustry/Prescriptions/ TheNon-MedicalPrescribingProgramme/ DH_099234)** and the NHS Education for Scotland website **(http://www.nes.scot.nhs.uk/education- and-training/by-discipline/pharmacy/pharmacists/ prescribing-and-clinical-skills/resources.aspx)**
PHARMACY TECHNICIANS	General Pharmaceutical Council **(www.pharmacyregulation.org)** 020 3713 8000	
DOCTORS	General Medical Council **(www.gmc-uk.org)** 0161 923 6602	To practise medicine in the UK, doctors are required to be registered with the GMC and hold a licence to practise
DENTISTS	General Dental Council **(www.gdc-uk.org)** 020 7167 6000	Dentists can legally write prescriptions for any medicine but they should restrict their prescribing to areas in which they are competent. Therefore they should, generally, only prescribe medicines that have uses in dentistry
		When prescribing on an NHS dental prescription, dentists are restricted to the medicines listed in the Dental Practitioners' Formulary (part 8a of the Drug Tariff for Scotland or part XVIIa of the Drug Tariff for England and Wales)

HEALTHCARE PROFESSIONAL	WHERE TO CHECK REGISTRATION	COMMON ISSUES
NURSES	Nursing and Midwifery Council **(www.nmc.org.uk)** 020 7333 9333	Nurses can have a range of further qualifications, which are annotated on the NMC register. Prescribing should be restricted to areas of clinical competence. Further information on non-medical prescribing, including FAQs, guidance and clinical management plans is available on the Department of Health website (National Archives) **(http://webarchive. nationalarchives.gov.uk/+/www.dh.gov.uk/en/ Healthcare/Medicinespharmacyandindustry/ Prescriptions/TheNon-MedicalPrescribing Programme/DH_099234)**
VETERINARY SURGEONS	Royal College of Veterinary Surgeons **(www.rcvs.org.uk)** 020 7222 2001	Veterinary surgeons can prescribe and requisition all human and animal medicines, including Controlled Drugs for the treatment of animals. Where Controlled Drugs are involved, these do not need to be on standardised forms Where the medicine is not licensed for the animal, then this needs to be prescribed under the veterinary Cascade (see section 3.6 for further details)
PARAMEDICS	Health & Care Professions Council **(www.hpc-uk.org)** 0300 500 6184	A Home Office group authority has been issued that allows paramedics to possess and supply certain Controlled Drugs under certain conditions. The Home Office has the authority to revoke or modify the authority at any time A full list of medicines that a paramedic can obtain for the purposes of administration is available on the MHRA website **(https://www.gov.uk/government/ publications/rules-for-the-sale-supply-and- administration-of-medicines/rules-for-the-sale- supply-and-administration-of-medicines-for-specific- healthcare-professionals)**

HEALTHCARE PROFESSIONAL	WHERE TO CHECK REGISTRATION	COMMON ISSUES
CHIROPODISTS OR PODIATRISTS	Health & Care Professions Council (www.hpc-uk.org) 0300 500 6184	Registered chiropodists and podiatrists can obtain additional qualifications that allow them to sell or supply and administer a larger range of medicines A full list of medicines that a chiropodist can sell, supply or administer is available on the MHRA website (https://www.gov.uk/government/publications/rules-for-the-sale-supply-and-administration-of-medicines/rules-for-the-sale-supply-and-administration-of-medicines-for-specific-healthcare-professionals)
PHYSIOTHERAPISTS	Health & Care Professions Council (www.hpc-uk.org) 0300 500 6184	
OPTOMETRISTS	General Optical Council (www.optical.org) 020 7580 3898	Optometrists can take further qualifications to become an 'additional supply optometrist' – this increases the range of medicines that they can sell or supply to patients (and therefore obtain a supply of from a pharmacy). A full list of the medicines that can be obtained is available from the MHRA website (https://www.gov.uk/government/publications/rules-for-the-sale-supply-and-administration-of-medicines/rules-for-the-sale-supply-and-administration-of-medicines-for-specific-healthcare-professionals) Further information on non-medical prescribing, including FAQs, guidance and clinical management plans is available on the Department of Health website (National Archives) (http://webarchive.nationalarchives. gov.uk/+/www.dh.gov.uk/en/Healthcare/Medicinespharmacyandindustry/Prescriptions/TheNon-MedicalPrescribing Programme/DH_099234)
DIETITIANS	Health & Care Professions Council (www.hpc-uk.org) 0300 500 6184	

HEALTHCARE PROFESSIONAL	WHERE TO CHECK REGISTRATION	COMMON ISSUES
ORTHOPTISTS	Health & Care Professions Council **(www.hpc-uk.org)** 0300 500 6184	Registered orthoptists who undertake additional training and obtain the relevant annotation on the Health and Care Professions Council (HCPC) register can sell, supply and administer certain medicines in the course of their professional practice. A full list of these medicines is available in Schedule 17 of the Human Medicines Regulations 2012 [SI 2016/186] as amended: **(http://www.legislation.gov. uk/uksi/2016/186/contents/made)**
RADIOGRAPHERS	Health & Care Professions Council **(www.hpc-uk.org)** 0300 500 6184	

3.4 Wholesale dealing

The Medicines and Healthcare products Regulatory Agency (MHRA) is the regulatory body with responsibility for oversight and enforcement of the wholesale of medicines. In July 2012 a regulatory statement issued by them (which was updated in March 2014) is in effect and has been reproduced in full with the permission of MHRA (**https://www.gov.uk/government/publications/repeal-of-wholesale-dealer-licence-exemption-for-pharmacists**).

MHRA STATEMENT

Guidance for pharmacists on the repeal of Section 10(7) of the Medicines Act 1968

With effect from 14 August 2012, Section 10(7) of the Medicines Act 1968 has been repealed. Section 10(7) provided an exemption in UK law from the requirement for a pharmacist to hold a Wholesale Dealer's Licence (WDA(H)) if they trade in medicines in certain circumstances. Its repeal was necessary in order to comply with EU legislation, in particular, Articles 77(1) and 77(2) of Directive 2001/83/EC which require anyone undertaking wholesale dealing activities to hold an authorisation.

This note provides guidance for pharmacists working in registered pharmacies and in hospitals on how MHRA, as the regulator responsible for the enforcement of EU legislation, will address the implications of the necessary repeal of Section 10(7) for the supply of licensed medicines by pharmacy other than direct to the public.

THE LEGISLATION GOVERNING SUPPLY OF MEDICINES

The legislation and underpinning guidance requires persons trading in medicines to hold a WDA(H) and to apply Good Distribution Practice (GDP) standards and have a suitably experienced 'Responsible Person' named on the licence to ensure that medicines are procured, stored and distributed appropriately. The legislation also ensures that medicines can only be supplied to other wholesale dealers, pharmacists or other persons authorised or entitled to supply medicines to the public. These rules also serve to provide confidence in the medicines supply chain by regulating the transit of medicines from manufacturer to patient.

HOW THIS APPLIES TO SUPPLY OF MEDICINES BY PHARMACY IN THE UK

MHRA is concerned to ensure that the repeal of the Section 10(7) exemption does not adversely impact on arrangements for supply of medicines in the UK. In determining how to address this issue, MHRA has taken careful account of the particular arrangements for delivery of healthcare in the UK which involve a wide range of individuals and in a diverse range of locations. In particular:

- *Many healthcare professionals and others authorised or entitled to supply medicines to the public in the UK need to hold small quantities of medicines for local healthcare provision and look to a local community or hospital pharmacy to supply them as part of their professional practice*

- *In contrast, some pharmacies engage in commercial trade in medicines, not solely as part of their professional practice within the UK healthcare system*

- *Pharmacists may also occasionally need to obtain small quantities of a particular medicine or medicines from another pharmacist in order to meet the needs of individual patients.*

MHRA ENFORCEMENT

MHRA takes the view that the supply of medicines by community and hospital pharmacies to other healthcare professionals in the UK who need to hold small quantities of medicines for treatment of or onward supply to their patients represents an important and appropriate part of the professional practice of both community and hospital pharmacy. Also community and hospital pharmacies may need to obtain small quantities of a medicine from other pharmacies to meet a patient's individual needs.

continued on next page

Both these activities are considered by MHRA to fall within the definition of provision of healthcare services. In such circumstances, provided the transaction meets all of the following criteria MHRA will not deem such transactions as commercial dealing and pharmacies will not be required to hold a WDA(H):

■ *It takes place on an occasional basis*

■ *The quantity of medicines supplied is small*

■ *The supply is made on a not for profit basis*

■ *The supply is not for onward wholesale distribution.*

Conversely, pharmacies who wish to engage in commercial trading in medicines are entitled to do so only if they hold a WDA(H) and comply with all the relevant requirements. As the authority responsible for enforcement MHRA will take appropriate action to enforce the requirement of the legislation and will require any commercial trade in medicines to be undertaken only by holders of a WDA(H).

These restrictions do not apply to the exchange of stock between pharmacies that are part of the same legal entity, although where a legal entity holds a WDA(H) as one (or more) of its pharmacies is involved in the commercial trade of medicines, the supplying pharmacy must also be named on the WDA(H) if the stock supplied is for the purposes of wholesale.

Guidance on the need for a WDA(H), the application process and a downloadable application form are available on MHRA's website.

http://www.mhra.gov.uk/Howweregulate/
Medicines/Licensingofmedicines/
Manufacturersandwholesaledealerslicences/index.htm
(applications)

http://www.mhra.gov.uk/Howweregulate/Medicines/
Licensingofmedicines/Informationforlicenceapplicants/
Licenceapplicationforms/Wholesaledealerslicences
applicationforms/index.htm (forms and guidance)

http://www.mhra.gov.uk/Howweregulate/Medicines/
Licensingofmedicines/Feespayablefortheregulationo
fmedicines/Feesforwholesaledealer'slicences/index.htm
(fees)

http://www.mhra.gov.uk/Howweregulate/Medicines/
Inspectionandstandards/GoodDistributionPractice/
Theinspectionprocess/index.htm
(the inspection process)

http://eur-lex.europa.eu/LexUriServ/LexUriServ.do?uri
=OJ:C:2013:343:0001:0014:EN:PDF
(Good Distribution Practice)

Please note: If you are making a supply outside of the scope of this regulatory statement you may be required to obtain a Wholesale Dealer's Licence (WDA(H)). Further information on the licence can be obtained from the MHRA (www.gov.uk/government/organisations/medicines-and-healthcare-products-regulatory-agency).

WHOLESALE DEALING OF CONTROLLED DRUGS

The Home Office and MHRA have advised that if a Wholesale Dealer's Licence (WDA(H)) is required, this also means that, if supplies include Controlled Drugs in Schedules 2 to 5 to the Misuse of Drugs Regulations 2001, then it is likely that a corresponding Home Office Controlled Drugs licence is also needed by the pharmacy to legalise this supply.

The following document 'Supplementary information on wholesale dealer and Controlled Drugs licences in the Health and Justice System in England' and the accompanying letter provide further information on this that is particularly relevant to pharmacists working in healthcare and secure environment settings. Please note that the requirements to hold Wholesale Dealer's and Home Office Controlled Drugs licences apply to all settings and not just those outlined in this document: **(http://www.rpharms.com/support-pdfs/2014-07-11--wdls-in-health-etc-settings---final-for-circulation-%283%29.pdf)** and **(http://www.rpharms.com/support-pdfs/2014-07-14-letter-re-supp-information-on-wdls-final-%283%29.pdf)**

PERSONS AND ORGANISATIONS THAT CAN RECEIVE MEDICINES

The range of persons and organisations that can receive medicines by wholesale is controlled by legislation and may also be restricted to certain medicines for certain purposes.

The full lists are extensive and beyond the scope of this document; however, Table 6 contains signposting information for persons who may commonly approach the pharmacy for medicines:

TABLE 6: SIGNPOSTING TO INFORMATION ON MEDICINES THAT CAN BE OBTAINED BY CERTAIN PERSONS

PERSONS	USEFUL REFERENCE SOURCES
MIDWIVES	MHRA. Rules for the sale, supply and administration of medicines for specific healthcare professionals (https://www.gov.uk/government/publications/rules-for-the-sale-supply-and-administration-of-medicines/rules-for-the-sale-supply-and-administration-of-medicines-for-specific-healthcare-professionals) Schedule 17 of the Human Medicines Regulations 2012 www.legislation.gov.uk Chapter 9, Dale and Appelbe's Pharmacy and Medicines Law. 10th edition. 2013
CHIROPODISTS/PODIATRISTS	MHRA. Rules for the sale, supply and administration of medicines for specific healthcare professionals (https://www.gov.uk/government/publications/rules-for-the-sale-supply-and-administration-of-medicines/rules-for-the-sale-supply-and-administration-of-medicines-for-specific-healthcare-professionals) Schedule 17 of the Human Medicines Regulations 2012 www.legislation.gov.uk Chapter 9, Dale and Appelbe's Pharmacy and Medicines Law. 10th edition. 2013
OPTOMETRISTS & ADDITIONAL SUPPLY OPTOMETRISTS	MHRA. Rules for the sale, supply and administration of medicines for specific healthcare professionals (https://www.gov.uk/government/publications/rules-for-the-sale-supply-and-administration-of-medicines/rules-for-the-sale-supply-and-administration-of-medicines-for-specific-healthcare-professionals) Schedule 17 of the Human Medicines Regulations 2012 www.legislation.gov.uk Chapter 9, Dale and Appelbe's Pharmacy and Medicines Law. 10th edition. 2013
PARAMEDICS	MHRA. Rules for the sale, supply and administration of medicines for specific healthcare professionals (https://www.gov.uk/government/publications/rules-for-the-sale-supply-and-administration-of-medicines/rules-for-the-sale-supply-and-administration-of-medicines-for-specific-healthcare-professionals) Schedule 17 of the Human Medicines Regulations 2012 www.legislation.gov.uk Controlled Drug Group Authority for paramedics (for morphine sulphate and diazepam) www.jrcalc.org.uk Chapter 9, Dale and Appelbe's Pharmacy and Medicines Law. 10th edition. 2013

PERSONS	USEFUL REFERENCE SOURCES
OWNER OR MASTER OF SHIP	Schedule 17 of the Human Medicines Regulations 2012 www.legislation.gov.uk
	Maritime and Coastguard Agency: Ships Medical Stores www.gov.uk/government/publications/msn-1768-applying-the-ships-medical-stores-regulations-1995 and list of corrections www.gov.uk/government/publications/msn-1768-corrigendum
	Chapter 9, Dale and Appelbe's Pharmacy and Medicines Law. 10th edition. 2013
ORTHOPTISTS	Schedule 17 of the Human Medicines Regulations 2012 [SI 2016/186] as amended http://www.legislation.gov.uk/uksi/2016/186/contents/made

Other persons or organisations that may obtain certain medicines include (please note this list is not exhaustive):

Doctors, dentists, any person conducting a retail pharmacy business, independent hospitals, clinics or independent medical agencies, first aid organisations, Royal National Lifeboat Institution and certified first aiders of this institution, occupational health schemes, Her Majesty's Armed Forces, drug treatment services, NHS Trusts. Schools may obtain salbutamol inhalers – see section 3.3.10.5 for further information.

Please note: Following discussions with the MHRA, our understanding is non-medical prescribers (e.g. pharmacist prescribers, nurse prescribers, etc) cannot receive a supply of medicines/wholesale of medicines within their own capacity (i.e. they are not listed in Schedule 22 or 17 of the Human Medicines Regulations 2012).

Schedule 22 of the Human Medicines Regulations 2012 (www.legislation.gov.uk) contains a full list of **persons and organisations** that are allowed to obtain medicines by way of wholesale.

Schedule 17 of the Human Medicines Regulations 2012 (www.legislation.gov.uk) contains a full list of **medicines** that persons and organisations can sell, supply or administer. They are able to obtain these medicines by way of wholesale.

Persons and organisations listed in Schedule 22 and 17 of the Human Medicines Regulations 2012 may also be able to obtain medicines from a pharmacy which does not possess a Wholesale Dealer's Licence (WDA(H)) if conditions outlined in the MHRA regulatory statement above are met.

SIGNED ORDERS AND RECORD KEEPING

When a POM is supplied from a registered pharmacy to healthcare professionals, an entry needs to be made in the POM register or the signed order/invoice needs to be retained for 2 years from the date of supply. Even where the signed order/invoice is retained, it is good practice to make a record in the POM register for audit purposes.

Schedule 17 of Human Medicines Regulations 2012 states which persons or organisations must provide a written signed order/invoice (one example is optometrists). For other persons or organisations where a requirement to have a signed order/invoice is not outlined in the legislation, we advise it is good practice to obtain a written signed order/invoice for maintaining an audit trail.

An entry in the POM register must include the:

■ Date the POM was supplied

■ Name, quantity and, where it is not apparent, formulation and strength of the POM supplied

■ Name and address, trade, business or profession of the person to whom the medicine was supplied

■ The purpose for which it was sold or supplied.

Legislation does not specify the details that need to be included on a signed order although local standard operating procedures (e.g. local NHS Trust policies or company SOPs) may require templates to be used. It would be advisable for the details required for a POM register entry (i.e. the list above) to be requested as a minimum for a signed order as this information would be required to complete the POM register.

See section 3.7.6 for details on the requisition requirements for Controlled Drugs.

If you are making a supply to persons or organisations under a Wholesale Dealer's Licence you will be required to follow Good Distribution Practice (GDP) **www.gov.uk/government/organisations/medicines-and-healthcare-products-regulatory-agency**

SUPPLY AND TRADE OF MEDICINES

The Department of Health has published a paper titled *Trading Medicines for Human Use: Shortages and Supply Chain Obligations;* this document has been endorsed by the RPS. This paper sets out the key legal and ethical obligations on manufacturers, wholesalers, NHS Trusts, registered pharmacies and dispensing doctors in relation to the supply and trading of medicines. Recent increases in the export of medicines are a major contributor to supply problems and risk jeopardising patient care.

The full paper can be viewed at **https://www.gov.uk/government/publications/trading-medicines-for-human-use-shortages-and-supply-chain-obligations--4**

Pharmacists can also consider information in the document titled *Best Practice Standards for managing Medicines Shortages in Secondary Care in England.* These standards are designed to provide advice to NHS hospitals in managing medicines shortages to minimise risk to patients. Please note: The principles apply to the rest of the UK but the document will require adapting for local structures in Scotland, Wales and N. Ireland.

These standards can be viewed at **http://www.rpharms.com/support-pdfs/managing-medicines-shortages-in-secondary-care.pdf**

FURTHER RESOURCES

Appelbe GE, Wingfield J, editors. *Dale and Appelbe's Pharmacy and Medicines Law. 10th edition.* London: Pharmaceutical Press; 2013.

MHRA. *Licences to manufacture or wholesale medicines.* **(www.gov.uk/government/collections/licences-to-manufacture-or-wholesale-in-medicines)**

MHRA. *Rules and Guidance for Pharmaceutical Manufacturers and Distributors 2015 – The Orange Guide.*

MHRA. *Rules and Guidance for Pharmaceutical Distributors 2015 – The Green Guide.*

Department of Health. *Supplementary Information on Wholesale Dealer and Controlled Drugs Licences in the Health and Justice System in England and accompanying letter.* July 2014. **(www.rpharms.com/support-pdfs/2014-07-11--wdls-in-health-etc-settings---final-for-circulation-(3).pdf)** **(www.rpharms.com/support-pdfs/2014-07-14-letter-re-supp-information-on-wdls-final-(3).pdf)**

3.5 Additional legal and professional issues

3.5.1 EXPIRY DATES

Where a product states 'Use by' or 'Use before', this means that the product should be used before the end of the previous month. For example, 'Use by 06/2017' means that the product should not be used after 31 May 2017.

Although the definition of 'expiry date' is less clear, the MHRA's advice to pharmaceutical manufacturers is: the term 'expiry date' should be taken to mean that the product should not be used after the end of the month stated. Therefore, an expiry date of 12/2016 means that the product should not be used after 31 December 2016.

3.5.2 WASTE MEDICINES

Information on the arrangements for disposing of pharmaceutical waste in England, Scotland and Wales is outlined in Table 7. For information regarding denaturing of Controlled Drugs, see section 3.7.10.

TABLE 7: WASTE ARRANGEMENTS IN ENGLAND, SCOTLAND AND WALES

For information regarding denaturing of Controlled Drugs, see section 3.7.10

	ENGLAND & WALES	SCOTLAND
ENFORCEMENT BODY	Environment Agency	Scottish Environment Protection Agency
CAN PHARMACIES RECEIVE WASTE MEDICINES?	Yes Generally, activities relating to waste require a licence. However, there are certain exemptions in place that allow these activities to occur without a licence. Some exemptions need to be registered while others do not. Under the Non-Waste Framework Directive (temporary storage at a collection point), pharmacies do not need to register an exemption to receive waste as long as the terms of the exemption are complied with. For further details see the Environment Agency website (**www.gov.uk/government/organisations/environment-agency**)	Yes The Waste Management Licensing (Scotland) Regulations 2011 allow registered pharmacies to accept returned medicines from patients or individuals and care services
SOURCES OF ADDITIONAL INFORMATION	Comprehensive information is available in a Department of Health publication entitled *Safe management of healthcare waste* (**www.gov.uk/government/organisations/department-of-health**) Other sources of information include the Environment Agency website (**www.gov.uk/government/organisations/environment-agency**) and the Pharmaceutical Services Negotiating Committee website (**www.psnc.org.uk**) – information specific to England but of use in Wales	Comprehensive information is available in a Department of Health publication *Safe management of healthcare waste* (**www.gov.uk/government/organisations/department-of-health**) and the Scottish Health Technical Note 3 Part B – NHS Scotland Waste Management Guidance: Waste Management Policy Template (**www.hfs.scot.nhs.uk**) Other sources of information include the Scottish Environment Protection Agency website (**www.sepa.org.uk**)
WHERE SHOULD WASTE MEDICINES BE STORED?	Waste medicines must be kept in secure waste containers in a designated area preferably away from medicines that are fit for use. If sharps are accepted, they should be stored in a sharps container	

	ENGLAND & WALES	SCOTLAND
DEALING WITH CONFIDENTIAL INFORMATION	Ensure that any patient identifiable information is destroyed or totally obscured	
TABLETS AND CAPSULES	Blister strips can be removed from their inert outer packaging but tablets and capsules should not be de-blistered. *(NB: An exemption applies to Controlled Drug tablets and capsules, which require denaturing – see section 3.7.10)*	
SHARPS	Dispose of syringes and needles in a sharps container	
LIQUIDS	The whole bottle (including empty bottles that may contain residue) should be placed into a pharmaceutical waste container because the mixing of different medicines could be hazardous. *(NB: Exceptions apply to Controlled Drug liquids, which require denaturing – see section 3.7.10)*	
ADVICE FOR PATIENTS	Patients should be advised that unused, unwanted medicines should be returned to a pharmacy for safe disposal	

3.5.3 COSMETIC CONTACT LENSES (ZERO POWERED)

Pharmacists who intend to sell cosmetic contact lenses (zero powered) need to consider the legal requirements within the Opticians Act 1989 and any subsequent rules and regulations that control the sale of such contact lenses. These products can only be sold under the supervision of a registered optician, dispensing optician or doctor.

FURTHER INFORMATION

The General Optical Council can be consulted on 0207 580 3898 (www.optical.org)

3.5.4 REQUESTS FOR POISONS AND CHEMICALS

Amendments to the Poisons Act 1972 have changed how poisons and some chemicals are classified and regulated. These require pharmacies to report suspicious transactions, significant stock loss and theft to the local police (dial 101) or the anti-terrorism hotline (dial 0800 789321). There is also a requirement for the public to present a valid licence issued by the Home Office before being able to purchase the most dangerous poisons or chemicals which could be used as explosive precursors. Where a licence is required, pharmacy teams will need to check that the licence is valid, unaltered and matches the request. Transaction details must be added to the licence, substances must be suitably labelled and regulated poisons require additional record-keeping in a poisons register. Where licences are not required, the pharmacist should

consider whether requests are suspicious and whether commercial alternatives or commercial retailers are appropriate to refer to.

Further information and details, including lists of regulated and reportable poisons and explosive precursors are available from the RPS guidance *Poisons and chemicals from pharmacy* (www.rpharms.com/support-resources/support-resources-a-z.asp).

Information on REACH (Registration, Evaluation, Authorisation & restriction of CHemicals), the CLP Regulation (Classification, Labelling and Packaging of substances and mixtures) and COSHH Regulations (Control of Substances Hazardous to Health) are available from the Health and Safety Executive (www.hse.gov.uk).

3.5.5 DELIVERY AND POSTING OF MEDICINES TO PATIENTS (INCLUDING ABROAD)

There are professional and practical considerations that are important when deciding whether or not to deliver medicines or whether or not to post medicines (prescribed or sold) to patients. The following are important to consider when making a professional judgement (the list is not exhaustive):

- Patient consent for delivery or posting
- Patient confidentiality during the delivery or posting process
- Whether it is necessary for face-to-face contact with the patient to ensure that the medicine can be safely, effectively and appropriately used
- Whether it is necessary to interview the patient
- Whether the patient has been assessed or directly interviewed by the prescriber
- Medicines and medical devices are not ordinary items of commerce and must be handled and supplied to the patient safely. An adequate audit trail must be in place for delivery and receipt from the point at which the medicine leaves the pharmacy and is received by the patient/patient representative or returned to the pharmacy in the event of delivery failure. Wherever possible a signature should be obtained to indicate safe receipt of medicines
- Storage requirements during transit
- When posting – will the postal carrier agree to transport the medicinal product (check terms of carriage, prohibited and restricted goods)
- When posting abroad – are there legal restrictions in the destination country which would prevent you from posting? (As an example, guidance produced by the U.S. Food and Drug Administration (FDA) makes it clear that it is illegal for a foreign pharmacy to ship prescription medicines that are not approved by the FDA to the United States)
- When posting abroad – are there UK legal restrictions which would prevent you dispensing in the first instance? (e.g. is the prescriber recognised as an appropriate practitioner (see 3.3.1) for the medicinal product in the UK?).

FURTHER RESOURCES

GPhC. *Guidance for registered pharmacies providing pharmacy services at a distance, including on the internet.* (**www.pharmacyregulation.org**) (see Appendix 13)

RPS. *Repeat medication management, prescription collection and delivery services.* 2015. (**www.rpharms.com/resources-AtoZ**)

Lists of internationally recognised narcotic and psychotropic drugs are available on the International Narcotics Control Board website (**www.incb.org**)

United States Food and Drug Administration (FDA). *Buying medicines and medicinal products online FAQs.* (Available under Drugs tab, resources for consumers **www.fda.gov**)

3.5.6 SECURE ENVIRONMENTS

Secure environments include prisons, police custody suites, secure hospitals, immigration removal centres and other places where persons are detained. Medicines and other health legislation may not refer specifically to the particular environment, and where this is the case then consideration should be given to best practice in either primary or secondary care, as appropriate, acting within the confines of the relevant legislation.

When medicines are dispensed from an 'in-house' pharmacy for administration or supply to patients within a prison, the pharmacy does not need to be registered with the General Pharmaceutical Council. Nonetheless, general pharmaceutical legal and good practice guidelines should be followed. If provision of a pharmacy service to another prison is being considered from an in-house pharmacy, advice should be obtained from the GPhC and MHRA to discuss whether the pharmacy premises would require registration or whether a Wholesale Dealer's Licence will be required.

The Secure Environment Pharmacists Group (SEPG) is a special interest group for pharmacists directly providing professional pharmacy and/or medicines management services to prisons or other secure environments. The SEPG provides an opportunity for networking and peer-level support and for the sharing of good practice.

> ## FURTHER RESOURCES
>
> Further information and resources for pharmacists working in secure environments can be found on the SEPG virtual network – accessible from the RPS website (**www.rpharms.com**).

3.5.7 CHILD-RESISTANT PACKAGING

Suitable, child-resistant packaging should be used for supplying all solid, all oral and external liquid dose preparations unless there is a good reason for not doing so. Such reasons may include:

- **SPECIFIC REQUEST** – the patient, carer or representative requests a packaging that is not child resistant, perhaps due to difficulty in opening it. The request may be met by supplying a non-child-resistant lid

- **ORIGINAL PACK** – the original pack may not be child resistant and there may be reasons underpinning why the medicine should remain in the original container. It may also be the case that no child-resistant packaging exists for a particular liquid medicine so it is not possible to change the container.

Where appropriate, the patient should be counselled to keep medicines away from the reach and sight of children.

3.5.8 REPORTING ADVERSE EVENTS

The role of most pharmacists involves contact with patients and receiving information from patients. Consequently they are in a prime position to identify adverse drug reactions. The Royal Pharmaceutical Society encourages, as a matter of best practice, the reporting of suspected adverse drug reactions under the Yellow Card scheme. Following a discussion with the patient, it may also be appropriate to make a record in the patient's notes and to notify the prescriber.

Reporting is possible online at **https://yellowcard.mhra.gov.uk**. Otherwise, a tear-out paper copy is available at the back of the BNF. A Yellow Card mobile app is also available though which side effects to medicines can be reported. The app also enables users to receive news updates from the MHRA.

The following two examples highlight the value of the Yellow Card Scheme and the importance of reporting suspected adverse events in this way. Warnings were added to the product information for varenicline after the MHRA received reports of suicidal ideation via the scheme and the Yellow Card reporting of adverse reactions to rimonabant (which was formerly used to treat obesity) contributed to the drug being withdrawn as new evidence meant the risks were considered to outweigh any benefits.

If a suspected adverse drug reaction (SADR) is related to a veterinary medicine which has affected a human and/or an animal, refer to section 3.6.

3.5.9 EMERGENCY CONNECTION TO EX-DIRECTORY TELEPHONE NUMBERS

Pharmacists can be connected to ex-directory, no-connection telephone numbers if they need to contact patients in a real emergency. This privilege is also available to doctors, hospitals and emergency authorities.

Pharmacists must use the privilege appropriately and only exercise their right of access when strictly necessary. The following guidelines must be adhered to:

- Pharmacists should only consider asking for connection to an ex-directory, no-connection number in a life or death situation. This can be interpreted as an emergency that is likely to pose a very serious threat to the health of a patient if information cannot be passed on immediately and when the patient's telephone number cannot be found from another source (e.g. the patient's GP surgery)

- A pharmacist needing to contact an ex-directory, no-connection number should dial 100, explain the situation and request connection to the number

- The pharmacist will only be connected when the following criteria are met:
  - The pharmacist explains the reason for the emergency connection request and advises the operator that it is a life or death situation (the operator will not judge the nature of the emergency but will accept the word of the pharmacist)
  - The pharmacist must give his or her name and the name of the pharmacy premises from which he or she is calling.

BT monitors all requests for emergency connection. If the privilege is abused it is likely that this important facility will be withdrawn.

3.5.10 HOMEOPATHIC AND HERBAL REMEDIES

Homeopathy has been defined as a holistic complementary and alternative therapy based on the concept of 'like to treat like' and involves the administration of dilute and ultradilute products prepared according to methods given in homeopathic pharmacopoeias.

Herbal preparations contain plant-derived materials, either as raw or processed ingredients which may be from one or more plants.

DIFFERENCES BETWEEN HOMEOPATHIC AND HERBAL PRODUCTS

The public can confuse homeopathic with herbal products as homeopathic products are often derived from herbs and are called by their botanical name, e.g. Aloe, and also because a single manufacturer may produce both homeopathic and herbal products. Pharmacists can help the public understand the difference between homeopathy and herbal products using information in our quick reference guide on *Homeopathic and Herbal remedies* (**www.rpharms.com/resources-AtoZ**).

EVIDENCE FOR HOMEOPATHY

There is no scientific or clinical evidence to support the efficacy of homeopathic products above the placebo effect, although anecdotal reports of their effectiveness have been published, particularly when used as part of individualised homeopathic treatment by a homeopathic practitioner. There is no evidence to support the clinical efficacy of homeopathic products beyond a placebo effect, and no scientific basis for homeopathy.

Given the lack of clinical and scientific evidence to support homeopathy, the RPS does not endorse homeopathy as a form of treatment.

ADVICE FOR PATIENTS

If a patient requests advice on homeopathy, the pharmacist should advise on the lack of evidence on the efficacy of homeopathic products, discuss the formulation and composition of the product, and provide advice relevant to the patient's condition. Pharmacists should also ensure that patients do not stop taking their prescribed medication if they take a homeopathic product.

REFERRAL

Pharmacists will be in a position to identify serious, underlying undiagnosed medical conditions requiring the patients to be referred to another healthcare professional.

Homeopathic products should only be used for the treatment of minor, self-limiting conditions, and must never be used for the treatment of serious medical conditions.

LICENSING

For the purpose of licensing, the MHRA does not currently require homeopathic products to demonstrate efficacy, only quality and safety. Further information about regulation of homeopathic products and registration is available on the MHRA website (**www.gov.uk/ government/organisations/medicines-and-healthcare-products-regulatory-agency**)

Herbal remedies must either have a full marketing authorisation based upon safety, quality and efficacy or a traditional herbal registration (THR) based upon safety, quality and evidence of traditional use. Further information is available on the MHRA website (**www.gov.uk/government/organisations/medicines-and-healthcare-products-regulatory-agency**)

FURTHER RESOURCES

RPS. *Homeopathic and herbal remedies – quick reference guide.* February 2010. (**www.rpharms.com/resources-AtoZ**)

RPS. *The traditional registration scheme – quick reference guide.* (**www.rpharms.com/resources-AtoZ**)

Williamson E, Driver S, Baxter K. *Stockley's Herbal Medicines Interactions.* 2nd Edition. London: Pharmaceutical Press; 2013.

Pharmaceutical Press. *Herbal Medicines.* 4th Edition. London: Pharmaceutical Press; 2013.

3.5.11 CHARITABLE DONATION OF MEDICINES

The World Health Organization in co-operation with major international agencies involved with humanitarian and developmental aid (including the International Pharmaceutical Federation (FIP), International Federation of the Red Cross and Red Crescent Societies) has published guidance (first edition 1996) that provides clear guidelines for the donation of medicine. We encourage any pharmacist considering donating medicines to read the document and adhere to the guidelines.

Pharmacists should be aware that if a pharmacy, in the course of its business, supplies a medicine to another business who obtains it for further supply, the supplying pharmacy will require a Wholesale Dealer's Licence (WDA(H))*. This is regardless of whether the medicine is stock surplus to the requirements of the pharmacy or general stock that is to be donated for charitable use or in times of conflict.

CONSIDER ALTERNATIVES

WHO encourages, in the acute phase of an emergency, that standardised health kits of medicines are donated. These kits are permanently stocked by major international suppliers such as Médecins Sans Frontières and the United Nations Children's Fund.

After the acute phase, WHO encourages the donation of cash that can be used to purchase essential medicines and is usually more useful than donations of medicines. Pharmacists and patients who want to help should be advised to donate money to charitable organisations to enable them to purchase supplies.

These cash donations may then be used by charitable organisations to obtain reduced price purchases from manufacturers (where available) who are able to supply suitable medicines for the target area, in appropriate quantities and with viable shelf life.

PATIENT RETURNS

The WHO guidelines specifically advise that patient-returned medicines should not be donated and describes these types of donation as an example of a double standard. This is because most countries do not allow the reuse of patient returned medicines within their own country. The WHO guidelines describe how these donations also frustrate management efforts to administer medicine stocks in a rational way and as a result, donation of patient-returned medicines is forbidden in an increasing number of countries. In the past, unsuitable medicines have been donated, leading to situations where stocks could not be used within their remaining shelf life and as a result the receiving country has faced costly and inconvenient destruction procedures. Most charitable organisations supporting the developing world or providing disaster or emergency relief will find it very difficult to use the miscellaneous collection of medicines that is received from the donation of patient-returned medicines.

Pharmacies accept patient returned medicines in the course of their business for destruction. MHRA has advised that if a pharmacy takes in a patient returned medicine and supplies it to another legal entity which then makes a further supply of the medicine, the pharmacy will be wholesale dealing the patient returned medicine. Wholesale dealing medicines requires a WDA(H)*. However, a condition of the licence provides that a medicine can only be obtained from a licensed manufacturer or wholesale dealer, or in the case of import from a non-EEA country for re-export to a non-EEA country, from a person in the non-EEA country who is complying with their local regulations. This condition therefore prevents the activity of taking in patient returned medicines for onward wholesale supply and reuse.

Articles 77(1) and 77(2) of Directive 2001/83/EC require anyone undertaking wholesale dealing activities to hold an authorisation.

REFERENCES

World Health Organization. *Guidelines for medicines donations* (3rd edition). Revised 2010. (www.who.int)

Regulations 18 and 44 of the Human Medicines Regulations 2012 [SI 2012/1916] as amended

SI 2012/1916 (http://www.legislation.gov.uk/uksi/2012/1916/contents/made)

SI 2013/1855 (http://www.legislation.gov.uk/uksi/2013/1855/contents/made)

3.5.12 ELECTRONIC CIGARETTES

Electronic cigarettes resemble cigarettes and deliver nicotine to the user via inhalation.

In June 2013, the MHRA confirmed that all unlicensed nicotine-containing products (NCPs), such as electronic cigarettes, are to be regulated as over-the-counter medicines to ensure public confidence in the safety and quality of these products. Further details can be viewed on the MHRA website.

The MHRA conducted scientific research into the safety and quality of existing products on the market and found that their quality varied considerably and hence described them as 'not good enough' to meet the public health priority of reducing the harms of smoking and passive smoking.

The MHRA is encouraging manufacturers of unlicensed NCPs to apply for a marketing authorisation.

The RPS supports the use of NCPs that have marketing authorisations; this would include where a manufacturer has obtained a marketing authorisation for their electronic cigarettes.

The RPS cannot endorse the use of unlicensed electronic cigarettes or other unlicensed NCPs. There is a risk of misleading patients that they are equivalent to licensed medicinal products.

Medicines which hold a marketing authorisation benefit from assurance of quality, safety, efficacy and from processes underpinned by Good Manufacturing Practice (GMP). NCPs that do not have a marketing authorisation do not benefit from the same quality control processes.

The RPS has a position statement on electronic cigarettes (www.rpharms.com/what-s-happening-/policy.asp). It was published in February 2014 after examining the currently available evidence on the safety and efficacy of electronic cigarettes and in light of current media and advertising campaigns by tobacco and electronic cigarette manufacturers.

REFERENCES AND FURTHER READING

GPhC. *GPhC outlines position on sale of e-cigarettes in registered pharmacies.* (www.pharmacyregulation.org)

MHRA. (National Archives). *Nicotine Containing Products.* (http://webarchive.nationalarchives. gov.uk/20141205150130/http://www. mhra.gov.uk/Safetyinformation/ Generalsafetyinformationandadvice/Product-specificinformationandadvice/Product-specificinf ormationandadvice%E2%80%93M%E2%80%93T/ Nicotinecontainingproducts/index.htm)

MHRA. *E-cigarettes: Regulations for consumer products.* 2016. (www.gov.uk/government/ organisations/medicines-and-healthcare-products-regulatory-agency)

3.5.13 COLLECTION AND PURCHASE OF MEDICINES BY CHILDREN

Pharmacists may be asked to supply dispensed medicines or to make sales or supplies of P or GSL medicines to a child/young person for themselves, on behalf of another person, such as a parent, other relative or neighbour or for persons whom they care for (this could be a parent or relative, etc).

It may be appropriate for a child to purchase P or GSL medicines for themselves or to register for the Minor Ailment Service where it exists, for example a young girl with period pain. Pharmacists should also be mindful of situations where requests for medicines may be linked to abuse. Further information on protecting children and young people is given in section 3.5.14 below, and on requests from children for oral emergency contraceptives as P medicines in section 3.2.2.

The decision on whether a supply or sale is appropriate will need to be dealt with on a case-by-case basis and will involve considering the individual circumstances. Sometimes there will not be a clear right or wrong decision, and different pharmacists with the same facts will make different choices. Whatever your decision, you should be prepared to justify this and make records of decisions where appropriate.

If in doubt, the following are some of the factors the pharmacist may want to consider when deciding whether the supply is appropriate or not. It is not possible for this list to be exhaustive.

1. **KNOWLEDGE OF THE CHILD:** Is the child known to the pharmacy? What information is known?

2. **MATURITY OF THE CHILD:** Is the pharmacist satisfied the child is capable and competent to understand the importance of the medicines they are collecting and are you satisfied there are no further concerns with them delivering the medicines. If the medicine is prescribed for the child, and the child is competent then patient confidentiality applies (see Appendix 4).

3. **NATURE OF THE MEDICINE(S) SUPPLIED:** What are the medicines being collected or supplied? Is there any applicable misuse potential? An example of this could be the sale or supply of laxatives which may be abused in anorexia. Is the pharmacist confident the child will not misuse or tamper with the medicine?

4. **PRIOR ARRANGEMENT:** Does the child regularly collect medicines from the pharmacy? Is the collection or purchase by the child pre-arranged by the patient? For example, an advance phone call by the patient or a letter of explanation.

5. **REASON FOR COLLECTION:** Is there a persuasive reason behind why the child is collecting or purchasing the medicine in the circumstances? For example, is collection on behalf of a patient who has mobility problems, is the child expected to self-medicate such as with an inhaler, is the child/young person a carer for the patient?

6. **COUNSELLING:** Does the patient require counselling? How will this be given? If the patient is the child, are they able to understand and fully competent?

7. **LOCAL POLICIES:** Are there any local policies which you should consider in your pharmacy or your local area?

8. **PROOF OF IDENTITY:** In some circumstances, such as with the supply of Schedule 2 Controlled Drugs, the pharmacist will usually ask to see identification of the collecting patient or representative. Children may not have ID to show and professional judgement can be used to decide if a supply is appropriate without identification.

FURTHER INFORMATION

Carers Trust provides support for young carers – further information can be found on their website (**www.carers.org**)

3.5.14 PROTECTING CHILDREN AND YOUNG PEOPLE

Pharmacists have a professional, legal and moral duty to protect children from abuse or neglect and to work with other organisations and authorities to safeguard children.

The following points may help with recognising signs of abuse or neglect; however, the list is not exhaustive and a series of minor factors could also be indicative of child abuse or neglect:

- **PHYSICAL ABUSE** – unusual/unexplained injuries, injuries in inaccessible places, bite marks, scalds, fingertip bruising, fractures, repeated injuries, age of injuries inconsistent with account given by adult, injuries blamed on siblings

- **NEGLECT** – poor growth and weight. Poor hygiene, dirty and unkempt. Inappropriate food or drink

- **EMOTIONAL ABUSE** – evidence of self-harm/self mutilation. Behavioural problems. Inappropriate verbal abuse. Fear of adults or a certain adult

- **SEXUAL ABUSE** – indication of sexually transmitted disease. Evidence of sexual activity or relationship that is inappropriate to the child's age or competence

- **PARENT/CARER SIGNS** – delays seeking medical treatment or advice and/or reluctant to allow treatment. Detachment from the child. Lacks concern at the severity or extent of injury. Reluctant to give information. Aggressive towards child or children.

If child abuse is suspected, you should follow local child protection procedures where these are available. If not, the process outlined in Diagram 8 may be useful.

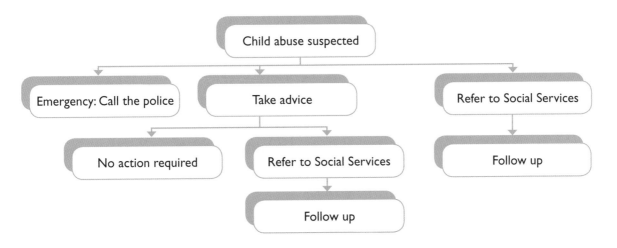

DIAGRAM 8: WHAT TO DO IF CHILD ABUSE IS SUSPECTED

Where you consider the nature of the child abuse to be an emergency then the police should be contacted.

Otherwise make a decision on next steps such as referring to local Social Services where appropriate or taking further advice. You should feel comfortable with sharing concerns and suspicions of abuse, even where these are not proven facts with Social Services.

You should not attempt to investigate suspicions or allegations of abuse directly.

You should make appropriate records of concerns and suspicions, decisions taken and reasons whether or not further action was taken on a particular occasion.

SEXUAL ACTIVITY IN CHILDREN

Children under the age of 13 are legally too young to consent to any sexual activity. Instances should be treated seriously with a presumption that the case should be reported to Social Services, unless there are exceptional circumstances backed by documented reasons for not sharing information.

Sexual activity with children under the age of 16 is also an offence but may be consensual. The law is not intended to prosecute mutually agreed sexual activity between young people of a similar age, unless it involves abuse or exploitation.

You can provide contraception (e.g. on prescription or under PGD) or sexual health advice to a child under 16 and the general duty of patient confidentiality applies, so consent should be sought whenever possible prior to disclosing patient information. This duty is not absolute and information may be shared if you judge on a case-by-case basis that sharing is in the child's best interest (e.g. to prevent harm to the child or where the child's welfare overrides the need to keep information confidential).

Remember that it is possible to seek advice from experts without disclosing identifiable details of a child and breaking patient confidentiality – and that where there is a decision to share information, this should be proportionate.

FURTHER INFORMATION

RPS. *Protecting children and young people – a quick reference guide.* 2011. (**www.rpharms.com/resources-AtoZ**)

3.5.15 PROTECTING VULNERABLE ADULTS

Pharmacists have a professional, social and moral duty to protect vulnerable adults from abuse or neglect and to work with other organisations and authorities to

safeguard vulnerable adults. The vulnerable adult's wishes should be taken into account at all times as a key issue is patient consent.

Vulnerable adults are persons who are over the age of 18 and are at a greater risk of abuse or neglect. They may fall into one of the following groups:

- Suffers from mental or physical disability
- Has learning difficulties
- Is frail or elderly
- Is in an abusive relationship
- Is a substance misuser.

Be aware that any of our patients, including those who do not fall within the groups above, could be a vulnerable adult. There are various types of abuse or neglect and the following lists may be helpful but are not exhaustive. The presence of one or more of these signs may not necessarily be caused by abuse or neglect.

- **PHYSICAL ABUSE** – injuries which are unusual or unexplained. Bite marks, scalds, fingertip bruising, fractures. Repeated injury
- **NEGLECT** – failure to thrive – evidence of malnourishment. Poor hygiene, dirty and unkempt
- **EMOTIONAL ABUSE** – evidence of self-harm/self-mutilation. Inappropriate verbal abuse. Fear of certain people

- **SEXUAL ABUSE AND RAPE** – indication of sexually transmitted disease. Repeated requests for emergency hormonal contraception
- **FINANCIAL ABUSE** – sudden changes to their finances, e.g. getting into debt. Inappropriate, exploitative or excessive control over the finances of the vulnerable adult
- **ADDITIONAL PERPETRATOR SIGNS** – delays seeking medical treatment or advice and/or reluctant to allow treatment of the vulnerable adult. Detachment from the vulnerable adult. Lacks concern at the severity or extent of injury or other signs. Is reluctant to give information. Aggressive towards the vulnerable adult.

Local procedures may be available from your employer, the NHS trust, Health Board or local council, and you should follow these procedures where available when abuse or neglect is suspected.

The process outlined in Diagram 9 below may also be useful.

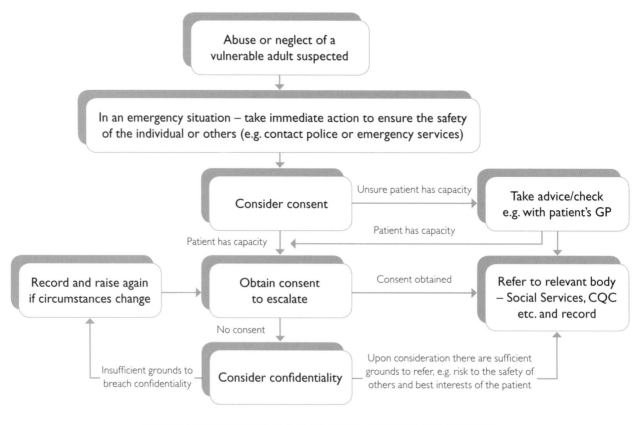

DIAGRAM 9: WHAT TO DO IF ABUSE OR NEGLECT IS SUSPECTED

A vulnerable adult's wishes should be taken into account at all times. Obtain consent from the patient before disclosing confidential information about them. However, if there are overriding circumstances requiring you to take immediate action to ensure the safety of the individual or others the need for referral, even if they do not give consent, should be considered. If you are unsure of someone's mental capacity to provide consent seek additional advice, e.g. from their GP.

You should not attempt to investigate suspicions or allegations of abuse directly or to discuss concerns with the alleged perpetrator of the abuse or neglect.

You should make appropriate records of concerns and suspicions, decisions taken and reasons whether or not further action was taken on a particular occasion.

FURTHER INFORMATION

RPS. *Protecting Vulnerable Adults – a quick reference guide.* 2011. **(www.rpharms.com/resources-AtoZ)**

Department of Health. *Mental Health Act 1983: Code of practice.* 2015. **(https://www.gov.uk/government/publications/code-of-practice-mental-health-act-1983)**

NHS Wales. *Mental Health Act 1983: Code of practice for Wales.* 2008. **(http://www.wales.nhs.uk/sites3/home.cfm?orgid=816)**

The Scottish Government. *Mental Health (Care and Treatment) (Scotland) Act 2003: Code of practice.* 2005. **(http://www.gov.scot/Topics/Health/Services/Mental-Health/Law/Code-of-Practice)**

3.5.16 MEDICAL DEVICES

A medical device is *any instrument, apparatus, appliance, material or other article, whether used alone or in combination, including the software necessary for its proper application intended by the manufacturer to be used on human beings for the purpose of:*

- *diagnosis, prevention, monitoring, treatment or alleviation of disease*
- *diagnosis, monitoring, treatment, or alleviation of or compensation for an injury or handicap*
- *investigation, replacement or modification of the anatomy or of a physiological process*
- *control of conception*

and which does not achieve its principal intended action in or on the human body by pharmacological, immunological or metabolic means, but which may be assisted in its function by such means.

Examples of medical devices (not exhaustive) available from a pharmacy include dressings, thermometers, needles, syringes, blood pressure monitor, stoma care products, condoms, test kits (e.g. cholesterol test kits, pregnancy test kits, etc.), inhalers, glucose meters and test strips, screening tests, some emollients, some eye drops, etc.

All medical devices are regulated by the Medicines and Healthcare products Regulatory Agency (MHRA).

All devices are required to carry the CE mark denoting compliance with the medical devices regulations and indicating that the device performs as intended, is fit for purpose with all associated risks reduced as far as possible.

FURTHER INFORMATION

RPS. *Medical devices – quick reference guide.* 2012. **(www.rpharms.com/resources-AtoZ)**

RPS. *Professional guidance for the procurement and supply of specials.* 2015. Includes guidance and case study on medical devices. **(www.rpharms.com/resources-AtoZ)**

MHRA. *Information on regulation of medical devices.* **(www.gov.uk/government/organisations/medicines-and-healthcare-products-regulatory-agency)**

MHRA. *Medical device education.* **(www.gov.uk/government/organisations/medicines-and-healthcare-products-regulatory-agency)**

MHRA. *Reporting adverse incidents involving medical devices.* **(www.gov.uk/government/organisations/medicines-and-healthcare-products-regulatory-agency)**

General Medical Council. *Good practice in prescribing and managing medicines and devices.* 2013. **(www.gmc-uk.org)**

NHS England and MHRA. *Patient safety alert. Improving medical device incident reporting and learning.* 2014. **(www.england.nhs.uk)**

3.5.17 ADMINISTRATION OF ADRENALINE IN AN EMERGENCY

WHAT IS ADRENALINE?

Adrenaline is a prescription only medicine and is given intramuscularly for the treatment of anaphylaxis. Brands of adrenaline intramuscular injections in your pharmacy may include Epipen®, Emerade® and Jext®.

Where a pharmacist is expected to recognise and treat an anaphylactic reaction as part of their usual clinical role (for example, if they are offering a vaccination service), they must have access to an anaphylaxis pack (as outlined in the Green Book) and have received the required training in the recognition of anaphylaxis and administration of adrenaline. The anaphylaxis pack will include ampoules of adrenaline and syringes and needles or prefilled syringes which should be used preference to auto injectors such as those listed above.

WHAT IS ANAPHYLAXIS?

Anaphylaxis is a severe, life-threatening, systemic hypersensitivity reaction resulting in rapidly developing airway and/or breathing difficulty and/or hypotension.

Other features of an allergic reaction are often present, including skin and mucosal changes such as urticaria and angio-oedema of the face. Anaphylaxis is an emergency which should be treated immediately once identified.

ADMINISTRATION OF ADRENALINE

Regulation 238 of the Human Medicines Regulations 2012 allows adrenaline to be administered by anyone for the purpose of saving life in an emergency (for further information see section 3.3.8).

Therefore pharmacists using their professional and clinical judgement can administer adrenaline in an emergency to persons presenting with symptoms of anaphylaxis.

If a pharmacist administers adrenaline they must also ensure that an ambulance is called by dialling 999 and reporting that there is a case of suspected anaphylaxis.

British National Formulary. (www.medicines complete.com or www.evidence.nhs.uk)

Human Medicines Regulations 2012. **(www.legislation.gov.uk)**

Section 3.3.8 of MEP 38. **(www.rpharms.com/resources-AtoZ NICE.** *CG134 Anaphylaxis.* 2011. **(www.nice.org.uk)**

Allergy UK **(www.allergyuk.org)**

Anaphylaxis campaign. (www.anaphylaxis.org.uk)

Public Health England. *The Green Book: Immunisation against infectious diseases – Chapter 8.* **(https://www.gov.uk/government/collections/immunisation-against-infectious-disease-the-green-book)**

Resuscitation Council (UK). *Emergency treatment of anaphylactic reactions: Guidelines for healthcare providers.* **(https://www.resus.org.uk/anaphylaxis/)**

3.5.18 MULTI-COMPARTMENT COMPLIANCE AIDS

Although multi-compartment compliance aids (MCA), (also known as monitored dosage systems (MDS)) may be of value to help some patients with problems managing their medicines and maintaining independent healthy living, they are one option following a comprehensive assessment of a patient's ability to safely manage their medicines. They may not be the best intervention for everyone and many alternative interventions are available. Evidence indicates that MCA should not automatically be the intervention of choice for all patients.

Not all medicines are suitable for inclusion in MCA and pharmacists should be aware that the re-packaging of medicines from a manufacturer's original packaging may often be unlicensed and involves risks and responsibility for decisions made.

With the limited evidence base currently indicating a lack of patient benefit outcomes with the use of MCA, it is a recommendation of the RPS that the use of original packs of medicines, supported by appropriate pharmaceutical care, should be the preferred intervention for the supply of medicines in the absence of a specific need identified by individual assessment for a MCA in all settings.

The RPS has published a repository of MCA information where key resources can be accessed including patient assessment tools and our guidance *Improving patient outcomes: The better use of multi-compartment compliance aids.* This can be viewed on our website at **www.rpharms.com/unsecure-support-resources/improving-patient-outcomes-through-the-better-use-of-mcas.asp.**

Pharmacists are encouraged to be aware of the risks associated with MCA use on a population basis without individual assessments, to be aware of the alternatives and to share this knowledge with other health and social care professionals.

UK Medicines Information has developed a Medicines Compliance Aid database that can be accessed by all pharmacists via the UKMi website at **www.ukmi.nhs.uk.** The database makes recommendations on the suitability of solid dose forms for transfer from the manufacturers' original packaging to MCA and should be used alongside the RPS Guidance.

UNDERPINNING KNOWLEDGE – LEGISLATION AND PROFESSIONAL ISSUES

3.5.19 DRUGS AND DRIVING

BACKGROUND

Section 4 of the Road Traffic Act 1988 includes an offence of driving whilst impaired through drugs, regardless of whether or not the drugs are being used legitimately. This means that if a patient's driving is found to be impaired by medicines, even if he or she is taking them as prescribed or as recommended in the product information, he or she may still be prosecuted.

A new additional offence of driving with certain specified drugs in excess of specified levels came into force on 2 March 2015 in England and Wales. The legislation also provides for a statutory 'medical defence' for patients taking their medicines as prescribed or in accordance with product information.

Roadside drug screening devices use saliva to identify if a driver has taken one of the drugs listed in table 8, or a drug that is metabolised to one of these. The first group are commonly abused drugs for which low limits have been set, the second group consists mainly of licensed medicines that have a significant liability to be abused and the specified limits have been set higher than those for the first group.

To protect patients who may test positive for certain drugs as a result of taking medicines in accordance with advice from a healthcare professional or the patient information leaflet, the new offence has a statutory 'medical defence'. This may be raised at any point providing that the drug was:

- Lawfully prescribed, supplied or purchased over-the-counter, for medical or dental purposes; and

- Taken in accordance with advice given by the prescriber or supplier, and in accordance with any accompanying written instructions (provided these are consistent with any advice given by the prescriber).

Patient specific advice provided by a healthcare professional may sometimes differ from the general information given in the patient information leaflet of a medicine. In these cases, the advice provided by the healthcare professional may be used as a basis for the patient's statutory 'medical defence'.

Pharmacists should be mindful of any new medicines added to a patient's regime that may interact with their existing therapies, affecting the metabolism of one of the specified drugs. They should also be cautious if there is a developing medical condition that could increase the risk of side effects from a medicine (e.g. during the development of a serious illness with significant weight loss).

TABLE 8: SPECIFIED DRUGS

FIRST GROUP	SECOND GROUP
Cannabis (THC)	Clonazepam
MDMA (ecstasy)	Diazepam
Ketamine	Lorazepam
Methylamfetamine	Oxazepam
Cocaine (and a cocaine metabolite, BZE)	Temazepam
Lysergic acid diethylamide (LSD)	Flunitrazepam
Heroin/diamorphine metabolite (6-MAM)	Methadone
	Morphine
	Amfetamine

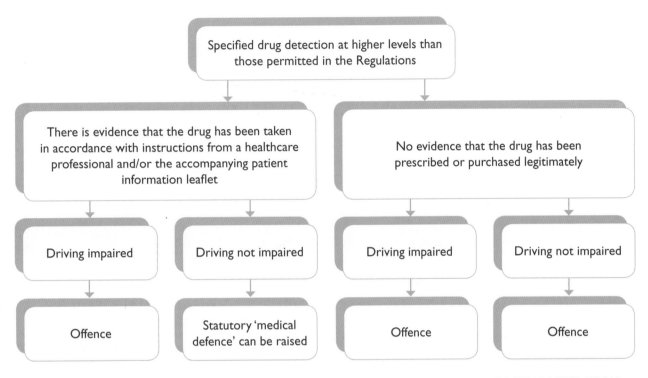

DIAGRAM 10: SUMMARY OF HOW THE NEW DRUG DRIVING OFFENCE FITS IN WITH EXISTING LEGISLATION

ADVICE FOR PATIENTS

Reminder of the advice that should be provided to all patients receiving medicines that may impair driving ability:

- You must not drive if you feel sleepy, dizzy, are unable to concentrate or make decisions, have slowed thinking, or if you experience sight problems. If the medicine is one that could affect your driving ability, you should not drive until you know how the medicine affects you as an individual, particularly when starting a new medicine or following a dose change

- If you start a new medicine, even if it is one that does not directly affect your driving you should check with your pharmacist if it could have an effect on any of the medicines you are already taking, that could in turn affect your driving

- Remember that alcohol taken in combination with medicines, even in small amounts can greatly increase the risk of accidents

- An untreated medical condition may itself cause driving impairment and so it is important that you do not stop taking your medicines.

In addition to this, patients who are taking medicines that are affected by the new legislation should also receive the following information and advice:

- There is new legislation in place which places limits on the amounts of certain drugs that you can have in your bloodstream whilst driving. There is a 'medical defence' for those who are taking medicines in line with a healthcare professional's advice, provided that their driving is not impaired

- Keep some suitable evidence with you when driving to show that you are taking your medicine as prescribed or supplied by a healthcare professional. Examples of evidence could include a repeat prescription slip for a prescribed medicine or the patient information leaflet for a P or general sale (GSL) medicine.

It is important to note that if the individual's driving is impaired, they can still be prosecuted under the existing offence of driving whilst impaired through drugs, for which there is no statutory 'medical defence'. It remains the responsibility of all drivers to consider whether their driving is or could be impaired by their medicines.

MEDICAL CONDITIONS AND DRIVING

In addition to the drugs and driving offences described in this section there are also rules on fitness to drive requirements for patients with certain medical conditions. Further information on medical conditions, disabilities and driving is available on the Driving & Vehicle Licensing (DVLA) website (**https://www.gov.uk/driving-medical-conditions**)

FURTHER INFORMATION

Information about whether a medicine is affected by the new legislation is included in its Summary of Product Characteristics which can be accessed via the **electronic Medicines Compendium www.medicines.org.uk/emc/).**

SI 2014/2868 *The Drug Driving (Specified Limits) (England and Wales) Regulations 2014* **(www.legislation.gov.uk)**

SI 2015/911 *The Drug Driving (Specified Limits) (England and Wales) (Amendment) Regulations 2015* **(www.legislation.gov.uk)**

Department for Transport. *Guidance for healthcare professionals on drug driving.* July 2014. **(www.gov. uk/government/publications/drug-driving-and-medicine-advice-for-healthcare-professionals)**

Perkins K. *Driving after taking drugs and medicines.* The Pharmaceutical Journal. 16 September 2014. **(www.pharmaceutical-journal.com/)**

Medicines and Healthcare Products Regulatory Agency. *Drug Safety Update. Drugs and driving: blood concentration limits to be set for certain controlled drugs in a new legal offence.* July 2014. **(www.gov.uk/drug-safety-update/)**

Medicines and Healthcare Products Regulatory Agency. *Drug Safety Update. Drugs and driving: clarification for Wales, Scotland, and Northern Ireland.* October 2014. **(www.gov.uk/drug-safety-update/)**

3.5.20 RETENTION OF PHARMACY RECORDS

Medicines Ethics and Practice refers to record keeping requirements throughout. In addition, East & South East England Specialist Pharmacy Services has published a document *Recommendations for Retention of Pharmacy Records*: **www.medicinesresources.nhs.uk/en/ Communities/NHS/SPS-E-and-SE-England/Reports-Bulletins/Retention-of-pharmacy-records/.** This document includes guidance for all pharmacy settings as well as some sector specific information.

FURTHER RESOURCES

Department of Health. *Records Management: NHS Code of Practice Part 1 and Part 2 Annex D1: Health Records Retention Schedule.* 2006. **(www.gov.uk/government/publications/ records-management-nhs-code-of-practice)**

3.6 Veterinary medicines

Pharmacists working in registered premises are authorised to supply veterinary medicines for use in animals under certain circumstances (e.g. when there is a valid prescription) and, as with human medicines, are responsible for any medicines supplied. There are various classes of veterinary medicines, which are summarised in Table 9.

TABLE 9: CATEGORIES OF VETERINARY MEDICINES AND THEIR CHARACTERISTICS

POM-V	Prescription-only medicines that can only be prescribed by a veterinary surgeon and supplied by a veterinary surgeon or a pharmacist with a written prescription
POM-VPS	Prescription-only medicines that can be prescribed and supplied by a veterinary surgeon, a pharmacist or a suitably qualified person on an oral or written prescription. A written prescription is only required if the supplier is not the prescriber
NFA-VPS	A category of medicine for non-food animals that can be supplied by a veterinary surgeon, a pharmacist or a suitably qualified person. A written prescription is not required
AVM-GSL	An authorised veterinary medicine that is available on general sale
EXEMPT MEDICINES UNDER SCHEDULE 6 OF THE VETERINARY MEDICINES REGULATIONS – EXEMPTIONS FOR SMALL PET ANIMALS (SAES)	An unlicensed veterinary medicine that does not require a marketing authorisation because it meets criteria laid out in Schedule 6 of the Veterinary Medicines Regulations - Exemptions for small pet animals. Further details are available in *Veterinary Medicines Guidance Exemption from authorisation for medicines for small pet animals* (**https://www.gov. uk/guidance/exemption-from-authorisation-for-medicines-for-small-pet-animals**)
UNAUTHORISED VETERINARY MEDICINE	An unlicensed medicine that does not have a marketing authorisation and is not eligible for exemption through the SAES. It can only be prescribed by a veterinary surgeon under the Cascade (see Diagram 12). This includes any human medicine used for animals

Prescription requirements for POM-V, POM-VPS and medicines supplied under the veterinary Cascade

The following must be present for a veterinary medicine prescription to be valid:

1 Name, address, telephone number, qualification and signature of the prescriber. Where Schedule 2 or 3 Controlled Drugs have been prescribed, the Royal College of Veterinary Surgeons (RCVS) registration number of the prescriber must also be included.

2 Name and address of the owner.

3 Identification and species of the animal and its address (if different from the owner's address).

4 Date; prescriptions are valid for six months or shorter if indicated by the prescriber (the Veterinary Medicines Directorate has confirmed in the case of repeatable prescriptions all supplies must be made within 6 months or shorter if indicated by prescriber). Prescriptions for Schedule 2, 3 and 4 Controlled Drugs are valid for 28 days.

5 Name, quantity, dose and administration instructions of the required medicine

NB: *The Veterinary Medicines Directorate advises that 'as directed' is not an acceptable administration instruction.*

6 Any necessary warnings and if relevant the withdrawal period (i.e. the time that must elapse between when an animal receives a medicine and when it can be used for food).

7 Where appropriate, a statement highlighting that the medicine is prescribed under the veterinary Cascade (e.g. 'prescribed under the Cascade' or other wording to the same effect).

8 Where Schedule 2 or 3 Controlled Drugs have been prescribed, a declaration that 'the item has been prescribed for an animal or herd under the care of the veterinarian' – usual Controlled Drugs prescription requirements apply (see section 3.7.7).

9 If the prescription is repeatable, the number of times it can be repeated.

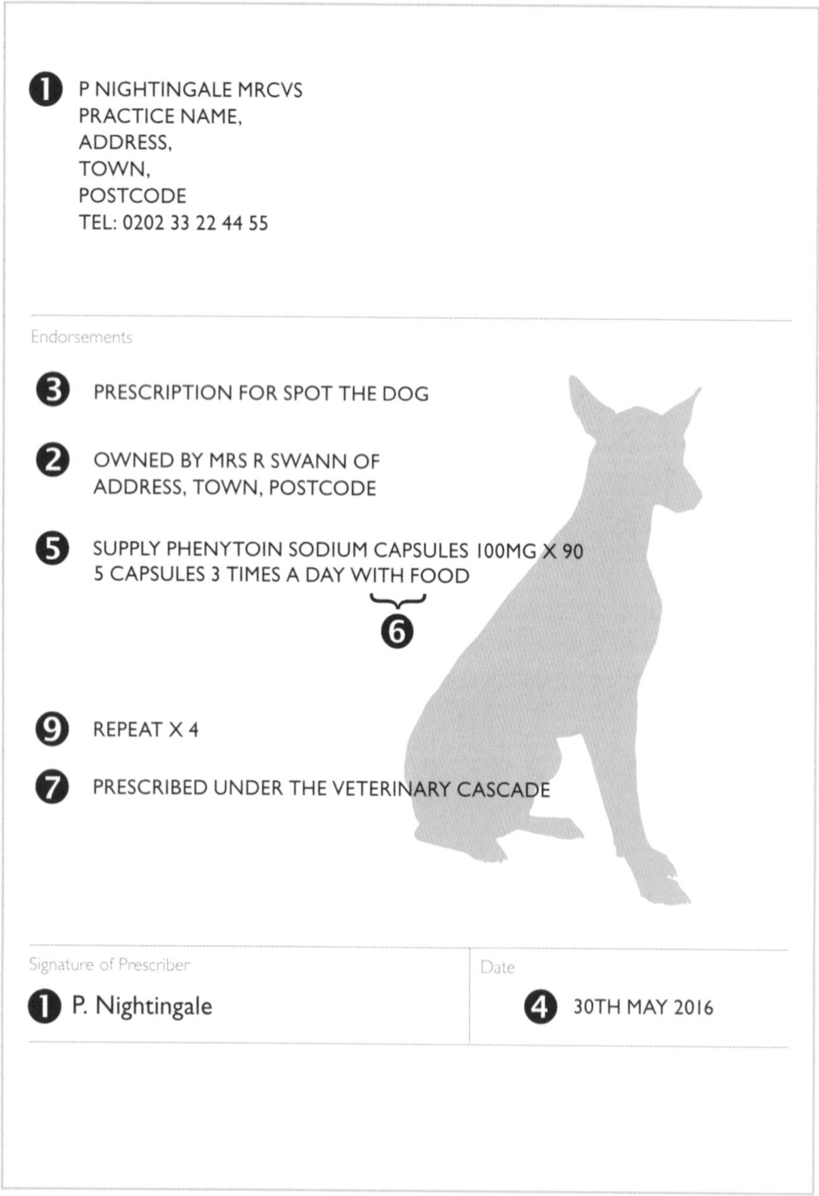

---

1 P NIGHTINGALE MRCVS
PRACTICE NAME,
ADDRESS,
TOWN,
POSTCODE
TEL: 0202 33 22 44 55

Endorsements

3 PRESCRIPTION FOR SPOT THE DOG

2 OWNED BY MRS R SWANN OF ADDRESS, TOWN, POSTCODE

5 SUPPLY PHENYTOIN SODIUM CAPSULES 100MG X 90
5 CAPSULES 3 TIMES A DAY WITH FOOD
6

9 REPEAT X 4

7 PRESCRIBED UNDER THE VETERINARY CASCADE

Signature of Prescriber
1 P. Nightingale

Date
4 30TH MAY 2016

DIAGRAM 11: VETERINARY PRESCRIPTION WITH CASCADE WORDING

TABLE 10: SIMILARITIES AND DIFFERENCES BETWEEN VETERINARY AND HUMAN CONTROLLED DRUG PRESCRIPTIONS

DIFFERENCES BETWEEN HUMAN AND VETERINARY PRESCRIPTIONS	SIMILARITIES BETWEEN HUMAN AND VETERINARY PRESCRIPTIONS
Standardised forms are not required for veterinary prescriptions; however, a statement that the medicines are 'prescribed for the treatment of an animal or herd under my care' is required for Schedule 2 and 3 Controlled Drugs. Standardised forms are required for human private prescriptions for Schedule 2 and 3 Controlled Drugs (see section 3.7.7).	Both are valid for 28 days from the appropriate date.

Usual Controlled Drug prescription content requirements (e.g. Total quantity in words and figures, etc. – see section 3.7.7) apply to both. |
Veterinary prescriptions should be retained for five years and not submitted to the relevant NHS agency. Original human private prescriptions for Schedule 2 and 3 Controlled Drugs must be submitted to the relevant NHS agency (see section 3.7.7).	
For all CDs, it is considered good practice for only 28 days' worth of treatment to be prescribed on veterinary prescriptions unless in situations of long term ongoing medication (e.g. when treating epilepsy in dogs). For human prescriptions the maximum quantity of Schedule 2,3 or 4 Controlled Drugs should not exceed 30 days. If more than 30 days is prescribed the prescriber should be able to justify the quantity requested (see section 3.7.7 under 'Total Quantity' for further detail).	
Veterinary prescriptions for Schedule 2 and 3 Controlled Drugs must include the Royal College of Veterinary Surgeons (RCVS) registration number of the prescriber. Human private prescriptions for Schedule 2 and 3 Controlled Drugs must include a prescriber identification number.	

The veterinary Cascade

A veterinary medicine with a UK marketing authorisation must be prescribed and supplied where one exists and is clinically appropriate. The Cascade exemption within the Veterinary Medicines Regulations allows the supply of medicines that are not licensed for animals. It is unlawful to supply a human medicine against a veterinary prescription unless it is prescribed by a veterinary surgeon and specifically states that it is 'for administration under the Cascade', or other wording to this effect.

NB: Although the wording on the prescription is a legal requirement, it is important that it reflects the actual Cascade (i.e. if a prescription is written generically for an animal with the Cascade wording present but a licensed veterinary medicine exists, then the Cascade requires the licensed product to be supplied rather than a medicine only licensed for human use).

The exemption specifies that where a licensed veterinary product is not available, other medicines can be considered as shown in Diagram 12.

Veterinary medicines licensed for another species, or for another clinical condition in the same species, extemporaneously prepared medicines or human medicines cannot be supplied against a veterinary prescription unless the prescription specifically states that it is *for administration under the Cascade*, or other wording to this effect.

Veterinary Medicines Guidance *The Cascade: Prescribing Unauthorised Medicines* advises that a human medicine may be used in accordance with the Cascade, assuming that the prescribing veterinary surgeon can justify the course of treatment based on animal welfare. Further detail of the Cascade and additional requirements for food producing animals is available in this guidance on the VMD website (**https://www.gov.uk/government/collections/veterinary-medicines-guidance-notes-vmgns**).

Where available it is a legal requirement to:

Supply a licensed veterinary medicine

Only where the above is not possible:

An existing licensed veterinary medicine for another species or different condition can be considered

Only where the above is not possible:

A licensed human medicine or an EU-licensed veterinary medicine can be considered

Only where the above is not possible:

Extemporaneous or specially manufactured medicines can be considered

DIAGRAM 12: VETERINARY CASCADE

Labelling

When a medicine is supplied by a pharmacy for use under the Cascade, the following details must appear on the dispensing label unless they already appear on the packaging and are not obscured by the dispensing label:

- Name of the prescribing veterinary surgeon
- Name and address of the animal owner
- Name and address of the pharmacy
- Identification and species of the animal
- Date of supply
- Expiry date of the product
- The name or description of the product or its active ingredients and content quantity
- Dosage and administration instructions
- If appropriate, special storage instructions
- Any necessary warnings for the user (e.g. relating to administration, disposal, target species, etc)
- Any applicable withdrawal period (i.e. The time between when an animal receives a medicine and when it can safely be used for food)
- The words: 'For animal treatment only'
- The words: 'Keep out of reach of children'.

Please note that the Royal Pharmaceutical Society recommends that the wording 'Keep out of the sight and reach of children' is included on the dispensing label.

If the medicine is not prescribed under the Cascade, the Veterinary Medicines Regulations do not specify that a dispensing label is required. However, the Royal Pharmaceutical Society advises that it would be appropriate to generate a dispensing label for all veterinary medicines, particularly for individual animals (pets).

Record keeping

The following points should be considered regarding record keeping for veterinary medicines:

- Records must be kept for receipts and supplies of POM-V and POM-VPS products and must show:
  - Name of the medicine
  - Date of the receipt or supply
  - Batch number
  - Quantity
  - Name and address of the supplier or recipient.
- If there is a written prescription, record the name and address of the prescriber and keep a copy of the prescription
- Pharmacists can either keep all documents that show the required information or can make appropriate records in their private prescription book
- Records can be kept electronically
- Records and documents must be kept for at least five years
- Pharmacies that supply POM-V and POM-VPS medicines must undertake an annual audit.

SALE OF UNAUTHORISED VETERINARY MEDICINES

It is unlawful to sell or supply unauthorised veterinary medicines (medicines not licensed as veterinary medicines), including human medicines such as general sale medicines (GSL) and P medicines, for an animal unless this takes place under the veterinary Cascade. This applies even if a veterinary surgeon asks the animal owner verbally to purchase an over-the-counter human product from a pharmacy.

SALE OF NFA-VPS AND POM-VPS MEDICINES

It is a legal requirement for pharmacists who supply NFA-VPS medicines or prescribe POM-VPS medicines to:

- Advise on how to use the product safely
- Advise on any applicable warnings and contra-indications on the packaging or label
- Be satisfied that the recipient intends to use the medicine correctly and is competent to do so
- Prescribe or supply the minimum quantity required for treatment.

PHYSICAL PRESENCE OF A PHARMACIST

Unless a transaction has been individually authorised in advance by a pharmacist and the person handing out the medicine is judged to be competent, the physical presence of the pharmacist is required for POM-V, POM-VPS and NFA-VPS medicines to be supplied.

ADVERSE REACTIONS

Pharmacists are increasingly supplying veterinary medicines for companion animals and should be mindful to the possibility that veterinary medicines can cause adverse reactions in humans as well as in animals exposed to a veterinary medicine. Suspect adverse drug reactions (SADRs) in humans are often associated with a failure to read and/or adequately follow product guidance information. Examples include animal sprays and 'spot-ons' onto human skin. The adverse reaction scheme for veterinary medicines is the equivalent of the 'yellow card' scheme for human medicines. Both animal adverse reactions and human adverse reactions to veterinary medicinal products should be reported. Details of the scheme and reporting forms are available at **https://www.vmd.defra.gov.uk/ adversereactionreporting/** or directly from VMD on tel: 01932 338427.

Wholesale dealing

VETERINARY MEDICINES

The Veterinary Medicines Directorate provides the following information in *Veterinary Medicines Guidance Retail of Veterinary Medicines.*

'*Only the manufacturer of a veterinary medicine or a holder of a wholesale dealer's authorisation (WDA) may routinely supply authorised retailers with veterinary medicines*'.

This guidance also states that '*An authorised retailer of veterinary medicines may supply products they are qualified to supply to another authorised retailer to relieve a temporary supply shortage, without a WDA. This exemption from the VMR is intended to prevent shortages of available medicines causing animal welfare problems. It is not intended to exempt wholesale supply from the need for a WDA.*'

Further information is available in *Veterinary Medicines Guidance Retail of Veterinary Medicines and Veterinary Medicines Wholesale Dealer's Authorisation (WDA).* **(www.gov.uk/government/collections/veterinary-medicines-guidance-notes-vmgns).**

HUMAN MEDICINES FOR VETERINARY USE UNDER THE CASCADE

The MHRA statement '*Guidance for pharmacists on the repeal of Section 10(7) of the Medicines Act*' that has been reproduced in section 3.4 also applies to the wholesale supply of human medicines to veterinary surgeons for use in animals under the Cascade.

The Veterinary Pharmacy Forum virtual network is available to members on the RPS website (**www.rpharms.com**)

Online resources, including a database of veterinary medicinal products and guidance documents are available on the Veterinary Medicines Directorate website (**www.gov.uk/government/organisations/ veterinary-medicines-directorate**)

Veterinary Medicines Directorate. *Veterinary medicines advice for pharmacists leaflet.* 2012. (**www.gov.uk/government/publications/veterinary-medicines-advice-for-pharmacists**)

The following two resources provide information on the legal requirements for the sale of veterinary medicines on the internet and the VMD Accredited Internet Retailer Scheme (AIRS):

Veterinary Medicines Directorate. *Sell veterinary medicines on the internet.* 2014. (**https://www.gov.uk/guidance/sell-veterinary-medicines-on-the-internet**)

Helping You to Buy Safe and Effective Veterinary Medicines on the Internet – the VMD's Accredited Internet Retailer Scheme leaflet. 2012. (**https://www.gov.uk/government/publications/accredited-internet-retailer-scheme-airs**)

National Office of Animal Health. *NOAH compendium of data sheets for animal medicines.* 2016. (**www.noahcompendium.co.uk**)

Details of a formal postgraduate veterinary pharmacy programme are available from the Harper Adams University website. (**www.harper-adams.ac.uk**)

Kayne S. *An Introduction to Veterinary Medicine.* Saltire Books; 2011.

Appelbe GE, Wingfield J, editors. *Dale and Applebe's Pharmacy and Medicines Law.* 10th edition. London: Pharmaceutical Press; 2013.

3.7 Controlled drugs

NICE. *Controlled drugs: safe use and management.* April 2016. (**www.nice.org.uk**)

*National Prescribing Centre (UK Web Archive). *A guide to good practice in the management of Controlled Drugs in primary care (England).* December 2009. (**http://www.webarchive.org.uk/wayback/ archive/20140627111322/http://www.npc.nhs.uk/ controlled_drugs/**)

*National Prescribing Centre (UK Web Archive). *Handbook for Controlled Drugs accountable officers in England.* March 2011. (**http://www.webarchive.org. uk/wayback/archive/20140627111322/http://www. npc.nhs.uk/controlled_drugs/**)

Appelbe GE, Wingfield J, editors. *Dale and Applebe's Pharmacy and Medicines Law.* 10th edition. London: Pharmaceutical Press; 2013.

Department of Health (National Archives). *Safer management of Controlled Drugs: a guide to good practice in secondary care (England).* October 2007. (**http://webarchive.nationalarchives.gov.uk/+/www. dh.gov.uk/en/Publicationsandstatistics/Publications/ PublicationsPolicyAndGuidance/DH_074513**)

National Treatment Agency. *Drug misuse and dependence: UK guidance on clinical management.* September 2007. (**www.nta.nhs.uk/guidelines.aspx**)

Ministry of Justice. *PSI 45/2010: Prison Service Order for Integrated Drug Treatment System.* September 2010. (**www.justice.gov.uk**)

NHS England. *Guidance for the handling of tramadol in health and justice residential sites.* June 2014. (**www. england.nhs.uk/commissioning/health-just/hj- resources/**)

Accountable Officers Network Scotland. *A guide to good practice in the management of Controlled Drugs in primary care – Scotland.* September 2014. (**www.knowledge.scot.nhs.uk/accountableofficers/ resources.aspx**)

The Scottish Government. *Safer management of controlled drugs: A Guide to Good Practice in Secondary Care (Scotland).* February 2008. (**www.sehd.scot.nhs.uk**)

NHS Protect. *Security standards and guidance for the management and control of Controlled Drugs in the ambulance sector.* Version 2. April 2013. (**www.nhsbsa.nhs.uk**)

NICE. *Managing medicines in care homes.* March 2014. (**www.nice.org.uk**)

Home Office. *Guidance for the safe custody of Controlled Drugs and drug precursors in transit.* September 2013. (**https://www.gov.uk/government/ publications/transporting-controlled-drugs- guidance-on-security-measures**)

Home Offfice. *General security guidance for Controlled Drug suppliers.* January 2014. (**https://www.gov.uk/government/publications/ general-security-guidance-for-controlled-drug- suppliers**)

Care Quality Commission. *The safer management of Controlled Drugs annual report.* (**www.cqc.org.uk/ content/controlled-drugs**)

Care Quality Commission. *Controlled Drugs governance self assessment tools.* (**www.cqc.org.uk/ content/controlled-drugs**)

These resources are archived and refer to The Controlled Drugs (Supervision of Management and Use) Regulations 2006 which have now been replaced by The Controlled Drugs (Supervision of Management and Use) Regulations 2013. The 2013 Regulations provide less detail of specific standard operating procedures and are focused on ensuring that adequate monitoring of Controlled Drugs is undertaken.

3.7.1 BACKGROUND

The core pieces of pharmacy legislation applicable to Controlled Drugs are:

- The Misuse of Drugs Act 1971 as amended (herein referred to as 'the 1971 Act')
- The Misuse of Drugs Regulations 2001 as amended (herein referred to as 'the 2001 Regulations')
- The Misuse of Drugs (Safe Custody) Regulations 1973 as amended (herein referred to as 'Safe Custody Regulations')
- The Health Act 2006
- Controlled Drugs (Supervision of Management and Use) Regulations 2013 which affect England and Scotland.

The 1971 Act imposes prohibitions on the possession, supply, manufacture, import and export of Controlled Drugs – except where permitted by the 2001 Regulations or under licence from the Secretary of State. The Safe Custody Regulations detail the storage and safe custody requirements for Controlled Drugs. The enforcement body for Controlled Drug offences is the Home Office, via the police.

The Health Act 2006 introduced the concept of an 'accountable officer' (see section 3.7.10) and requires healthcare organisations, and those providing services to healthcare organisations, to have standard operating procedures in place for using and managing Controlled Drugs.

For registered pharmacies, the Responsible Pharmacist Regulations 2008 also require that a range of pharmacy procedures are established – including procedures for Controlled Drugs (see Appendix 10).

Pharmacists should ensure that they are familiar with the standard operating procedures for managing controlled drugs in their pharmacies and the steps that they should take should an incident or concern relating to Controlled Drugs arise.

Accountable officers

Following the Shipman Inquiry, accountable officers were introduced with responsibility for supervising and managing the use of Controlled Drugs in their organisation or setting. Accountable officers have many roles and responsibilities These include:

- oversight of the monitoring and auditing of the management, prescribing and use of Controlled Drugs
- ensuring that systems are in place for recording concerns and incidents involving Controlled Drugs and the operation of these systems
- attendance of Local Intelligence Network meetings
- submission of occurrence reports which describe the details of any concerns the organisation has had regarding the management of Controlled Drugs in a required time frame
- the appointment of authorised witnesses for the destruction of Controlled Drugs.

Further information on the types of individuals who can become authorised witnesses can be found in the documents *The Controlled Drugs (Supervision of Management and Use) Regulations 2013 NHS England Single Operating Model* (**www.england.nhs.uk/publications/**) and *A Guide to Good Practice in the Management of Controlled Drugs in Primary Care – Scotland* (**www.knowledge.scot. nhs.uk/accountableofficers/resources-library/resource-detail.aspx?id=4055959**). Sources of further information on the duties of accountable officers are specified in Table 11.

TABLE 11: SOURCES OF INFORMATION ON THE DUTIES OF ACCOUNTABLE OFFICERS AND LISTS OF ACCOUNTABLE OFFICERS

ENGLAND	The National Prescribing Centre has published a document that describes the core role of accountable officers. The resource is entitled the *Handbook of Controlled Drug accountable officers in England (1st edition)* and is available on the UK Web Archive (**www.webarchive.org. uk/wayback/archive/20140627111322/http://www.npc.nhs.uk/controlled_drugs/**). NHS England have also published guidance The Controlled Drugs (Supervision of Management and Use Regulations 2013 NHS England Single Operating Model (**www.england.nhs.uk/publications/**) A register of accountable officers in England is published on the Care Quality Commission website (**www.cqc.org.uk**)
SCOTLAND	Information on the role of accountable officers and a list of accountable officers in Scotland is available on the Healthcare Improvement Scotland website (**www.healthcareimprovementscotland.org/our_work/governance_and_assurance/ controlled_drugs.aspx**)
WALES	Information regarding the role of accountable officers in Wales and a list of accountable officers is available on the Healthcare Inspectorate Wales website (**www.hiw.org.uk**)

3.7.2 CLASSIFICATION

The 2001 Regulations classify Controlled Drugs into five Schedules according to the different levels of control attributed to each:

■ Schedule 1 (CD Lic POM)

■ Schedule 2 (CD POM)

■ Schedule 3 (CD No Register POM)

■ Schedule 4 (CD Benz POM and CD Anab POM)

■ Schedule 5 (CD INV P and CD INV POM).

Information regarding the CD Schedule of medicines with monographs is available within the British National Formulary for Schedule 1 to Schedule 4 medicines. See also Section 6: Excluded topics and signposted for additional resources.

Schedule 1 (CD Lic POM)

Most Schedule 1 drugs have no therapeutic use and a licence is generally required for their production, possession or supply. Examples include hallucinogenic drugs (e.g. 'LSD'), ecstasy-type substances, raw opium and cannabis.

Schedule 2 (CD POM)

Pharmacists and other classes of person named in the 2001 Regulations have a general authority to possess, supply and procure Schedule 2 Controlled Drugs when acting in that capacity.

Schedule 2 includes opiates (e.g. diamorphine, morphine, methadone, oxycodone, pethidine), major stimulants (e.g. amfetamines), quinalbarbitone and ketamine.

Schedule 3 (CD No Register POM)

Schedule 3 Controlled Drugs include minor stimulants and other drugs (such as buprenorphine, temazepam, tramadol, midazolam and phenobarbital) that are less likely to be misused (and less harmful if misused) than those in Schedule 2.

Schedule 4
(CD Benz POM or CD Anab POM)

Schedule 4 is split into two parts:

■ Part I (CD Benz POM) – contains most of the benzodiazepines (such as diazepam), non-benzodiazepine hypnotics (such as zopiclone), and Sativex (a cannabinoid oromucosal mouth spray)

■ Part II (CD Anab POM) – contains most of the anabolic and androgenic steroids, together with clenbuterol (an adrenoceptor stimulant) and growth hormones.

Schedule 5
(CD INV POM or CD INV P)

Schedule 5 contains preparations of certain Controlled Drugs (such as codeine, pholcodine and morphine) that are exempt from full control when present in medicinal products of specifically low strengths.

Table 12 summarises the various characteristics of Controlled Drugs.

TABLE 12: SUMMARY OF VARIOUS CHARACTERISTICS OF CONTROLLED DRUGS

	SCHEDULE 2	SCHEDULE 3	SCHEDULE 4 (PART I)	SCHEDULE 4 (PART II)	SCHEDULE 5
DESIGNATION	CD POM	CD No Reg POM	CD Benz POM	CD Anab POM	CD INV P or CD INV POM
PRESCRIPTION REQUIREMENTS – SEE SECTION 3.7.7	Yes	Yes	No	No	No
PRESCRIPTION VALID FOR	28 days after appropriate date	28 days after appropriate date	28 days after appropriate date	28 days after appropriate date	6 months
ADDRESS OF PRESCRIBER REQUIRED TO BE WITHIN THE UK	Yes	Yes	No	No	No
EEA & SWISS PRESCRIBERS CAN LEGALLY PRESCRIBE	No	No	Yes	Yes	Yes
PRESCRIPTION IS REPEATABLE*	No	No	Yes	Yes	Yes

	SCHEDULE 2	SCHEDULE 3	SCHEDULE 4 (PART I)	SCHEDULE 4 (PART II)	SCHEDULE 5
EMERGENCY SUPPLY	No	No (except phenobarbital [also known as phenobarbitone or phenobarbitone sodium] for epilepsy by a UK-registered prescriber)	Yes	Yes	Yes
REQUISITION NECESSARY	Yes	Yes	No	No	No
REQUISITION TO BE MARKED BY THE SUPPLIER	Yes	Yes	No	No	No
INVOICES TO BE RETAINED FOR TWO YEARS**	No	Yes	No	No	Yes
LICENCE REQUIRED TO IMPORT OR EXPORT	Yes	Yes	Yes	Yes (unless the substance is imported or exported by a person for self-administration)	No

*By 'repeatable' we mean the instance where the prescriber adds an instruction on the main prescription for the prescribed item to be repeated, e.g. repeat x 3. This does not refer to the prescription counterpart which is sometimes used as a patient repeat request to the prescriber. NHS prescriptions are not repeatable (see section 3.3.1 under repeatable prescriptions).

**NICE advise that organisations should consider retaining all Controlled Drugs invoices for six years for the purpose of HM Revenue and Customs.

3.7.3 POSSESSION AND SUPPLY

Pharmacists, doctors and dentists, when acting in these capacities, are among those empowered by the 2001 Regulations under a general authority to possess, supply and procure Schedule 2, 3, 4 and 5 Controlled Drugs.

Other mechanisms for the lawful possession of Controlled Drugs include:

- **HOME OFFICE LICENCE** – persons who have an applicable Home Office licence can possess and supply Controlled Drugs in accordance with the terms of the licence (e.g. the museum of the Royal Pharmaceutical Society holds a Home Office licence to possess Controlled Drugs for the purposes of the museum)

- **HOME OFFICE GROUP AUTHORITY** – persons who are covered by an applicable Home Office licence group authority can possess and supply Controlled Drugs in accordance with the terms of the group authority (e.g. there is currently a group authority covering paramedics that allows them to possess and supply certain Controlled Drugs)

- **LEGISLATION: CLASS OF PERSON** – other classes of person specified in the 2001 Regulations, provided they are acting in the capacity of the specified class (e.g. a postal operator or, for specified Controlled Drugs, a registered practising midwife)

- **LEGISLATION: CLASS OF DRUG** – the 2001 Regulations indicate that possessing certain classes of Controlled Drugs is lawful (e.g. Schedule 4 part II drugs when contained in medicinal products and Schedule 5 drugs)

- **PATIENTS** – persons who have been prescribed a Controlled Drug by a doctor, supplementary prescriber, nurse independent prescriber, pharmacist independent prescriber, dentist or veterinary surgeon (for an animal).

A comprehensive analysis of the multiple classes of persons who, and organisations that, can possess and supply Controlled Drugs is outside the scope of this document. However, this has been summarised within Chapter 17 of *Pharmacy and Medicines Law* (10th edition. 2013) or can be found in the 2001 Regulations.

Possession of Schedule 1 Controlled Drugs

A Home Office licence would be required to possess Schedule 1 Controlled Drugs. However, some pharmacists, particularly those working within a hospital, may be asked to deal with substances removed from patients on admission, which may be Schedule 1 products (e.g. cannabis). A pharmacist, under two specific exemptions, can take possession of such Controlled Drugs. The first exemption is when possession is taken for the purpose of destruction. The second is for the purpose of handing over to a police officer.

The patient's confidentiality should normally be maintained and the police should be called on the understanding that the source will not be identified. If, however, the quantity is so large that the drug could not be purely for personal use the pharmacist may decide that the greater interests of the public require identification of the source. Such a decision should not be taken without first considering discussing the situation with the other health professionals involved in the patient's care and taking advice from the pharmacist's professional indemnity insurer's legal adviser.

The patient should give authority for the drug to be removed and destroyed. If the patient refuses, the pharmacist may feel that he or she has no alternative other than to call in the police. Under no circumstances can a suspected illicit drug be handed back to a patient.

3.7.4 ADMINISTRATION

Schedule 1 Controlled Drugs may only be administered, or prescribed under a Home Office licence.

Schedule 2, 3 or 4 Controlled Drugs can be administered to a patient by:

- A doctor, dentist, pharmacist independent prescriber or nurse independent prescriber acting in their own right

- A supplementary prescriber (including a pharmacist supplementary prescriber) acting in accordance with a clinical management plan

- A person acting in accordance with the directions of a prescriber entitled to prescribe Controlled Drugs (including pharmacist independent prescribers).

Since 23 April 2012, pharmacist independent prescribers have been empowered to be able to prescribe Schedule 2, 3, 4 and 5 Controlled Drugs, administer them in their own right or direct their administration.

Only medical prescribers who hold a special licence from the Home Secretary or Scottish Government's Chief Medical Officer can prescribe cocaine, diamorphine or dipipanone for treating addiction. This special licence is not required if treating organic disease or injury. Pharmacist independent prescribers, nurse independent prescribers and supplementary prescribers may not prescribe cocaine, diamorphine or dipipanone for treating addiction, but may prescribe these medicines for treating organic disease or injury.

NB: In healthcare environments, including secure environments, additional requirements and restrictions regarding who may administer or witness the administration of medicines may exist to satisfy medicines management, governance and patient safety considerations.

3.7.5 IMPORT, EXPORT AND TRAVELLERS

A licence is needed for a pharmacy to import or export Schedule 1, 2, 3 and 4 (part 1) Controlled Drugs. A licence is needed for Schedule 4 (part II) Controlled Drugs, unless the substance is imported or exported by a person for self-administration. There are no restrictions on the import or export of Schedule 5 Controlled Drugs (see Table 12).

Pharmacists are often asked about arrangements for patients who are taking Controlled Drugs abroad. The Home Office is the regulatory body in this instance and may require individuals to apply for personal licences in certain circumstances. Information can be found on the Home Office website **(www.gov.uk/government/organisations/home-office)**.

TRAVELLERS

At the time of writing, a personal licence was not required by the Home Office if a person travelling is carrying less than three months' supply of a Controlled Drug. However, it is advised that a covering letter from the prescriber is obtained that confirms the name of the patient, travel plans, name of the prescribed Controlled Drug, total quantities and dose.

The patient should also check with the embassies or high commissions for the countries they will be travelling through to ensure that the import and export regulations in those countries are complied with.

It would be prudent for patients to check any additional requirements that their travel operator/airline company may impose.

3.7.6 OBTAINING CONTROLLED DRUGS – REQUISITION REQUIREMENTS FOR SCHEDULE 1, 2 AND 3 CONTROLLED DRUGS

On 30 November 2015, amendments to the Misuse of Drugs Regulations 2001 made the use of an approved form for the requisitioning of Schedule 2 and 3 Controlled Drugs in the community mandatory. This applies to both requisitions for human and for veterinary use. Hospices and prisons are exempt from the requirement to use the approved form. The introduction of an approved mandatory requisition form is a remaining Shipman Inquiry recommendation aimed at ensuring the purchase of all stocks of Schedule 2 and 3 Controlled Drugs by healthcare professionals within the community can be monitored.

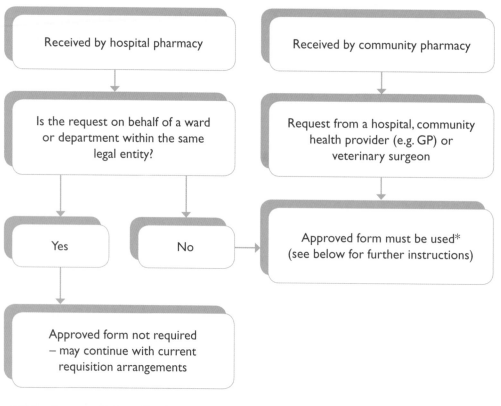

* Unless the request is from a hospice or prison

DIAGRAM 13: SUMMARY OF WHEN AN APPROVED MANDATORY REQUISITION FORM MUST BE USED TO REQUEST STOCK OF SCHEDULE 2 AND 3 CONTROLLED DRUGS

The handling of Controlled Drugs in prisons requires specific processes. In England these are underpinned by the information currently found in the NPC document (UK Web Archive) *Safe Management and Use of Controlled Drugs in Prison Health in England* (**www.webarchive.org.uk/wayback/archive/20140627111322/http://www.npc.nhs.uk/controlled_drugs/**).

In prisons in England, hospital-style requisition forms (instead of a standardised form) are usually used and are printed in a bound, book format – sequentially numbered with a carbon copy of each requisition to provide a robust audit trail. Although not a legal requirement, prisons in Scotland currently use standardised CDRF forms to request stock.

THE LEGAL REQUIREMENTS FOR A CONTROLLED DRUG REQUISITION ARE:

1. Signature of the recipient
2. Name of the recipient
3. Address of the recipient
4. Profession or occupation
5. Total quantity of drug
6. Purpose of the requisition

HOSPITAL REQUISITIONS

Hospital pharmacy requisitions from a ward or department that are presented to a pharmacy that is a separate legal entity must also meet these requirements, including the use of an approved mandatory requisition form. The Home Office has advised that the person in charge or acting in charge of a hospital can issue a yearly 'bulk' or 'global' requisition on the approved mandatory form to the separate legal entity that supplies its wards or departments for the wards or departments to then draw on throughout the year using Controlled Drugs requisition books with duplicate pages. The full Home Office guidance specific to this scenario can be accessed on the NHSBSA website **(http://www.nhsbsa.nhs.uk/PrescriptionServices/1120.aspx)**. Where the person in charge, or acting in charge of a hospital issues and signs a requisition, this must also be signed by a doctor or dentist employed or engaged in that hospital.

PRACTICE ISSUES

- Supplies made against a faxed or photocopied requisition are not acceptable

- Legislation requires that a requisition in writing must be obtained by the supplier (i.e. the pharmacy) before delivery of any Schedule 2 or 3 Controlled Drug to most recipients – including practitioners, hospitals, care homes, ship and offshore installation personnel, senior registered nurses in charge of wards, theatres and other hospital departments. Some recipients (such as GPhC registered pharmacies) are not included in this legal requirement. However, the Home Office advises that supplies from one registered pharmacy to another registered pharmacy should only be made after receiving a written requisition on an approved requisition form

- In an emergency, a doctor or dentist can be supplied with a Schedule 2 or 3 Controlled Drug on the undertaking that a requisition will be supplied within the next 24 hours. Failure to do so would be an offence on the part of the doctor or dentist

- Where stock is collected by a messenger on behalf of a purchaser, a written authorisation must be provided to the supplying pharmacist that empowers the messenger to receive the medicines on behalf of the purchaser. The supplying pharmacist needs to be reasonably satisfied that the authorisation is genuine and must retain it for two years

- A licence would be required for any healthcare professional to possess Schedule 1 Controlled Drugs; pharmacists are reminded that they are not able to requisition Schedule 1 Controlled Drugs

- For further details on wholesale dealing see section 3.4.

TABLE 13: APPROVED MANDATORY REQUISITION FORMS

	ENGLAND	SCOTLAND*	WALES
TYPE OF FORM	New style FP10CDF	CDRF – for private supplies GP10A – for NHS supplies	WP10CDF
WHERE TO OBTAIN FORMS	Download from NHSBSA website (www.nhsbsa.nhs.uk/PrescriptionServices/1120.aspx)	Local NHS health board	Local NHS health board

At the time of writing, in Scotland, the GP10A remains the main form required for the requisition of Controlled Drugs, with the exception of private supply. Further information on the requisitioning of Controlled Drugs in Scotland is available on the NHS National Services Scotland Practitioner Services website (http://www.psd.scot.nhs.uk/professionals/pharmacy/controlled-drugs.html).

PROCESSING REQUISITION FORMS (MARKING AND SENDING)

When a requisition for a Schedule 1, 2 or 3 Controlled Drug is received, it is a legal requirement to:

- Mark the requisition indelibly with the supplier's name and address (i.e. the name of the pharmacy); where a pharmacy stamp is used this must be clear and legible

- Send the original requisition to the relevant NHS agency.

As a matter of good practice, pharmacies should retain a copy of the requisition for two years from the date of supply.

These processing requirements do not apply when the supply is made:

- By a person responsible for the dispensing and supply of medicines at a hospital, care home, hospice, prison or organisation providing ambulance services who must mark and retain the original requisition for two years

- By pharmaceutical manufactures or wholesalers

- Against veterinary requisitions (the original requisition should be retained for five years).

Midwife supply orders

A registered midwife may use a midwife supply order to obtain the following Controlled Drugs:

- Diamorphine
- Morphine
- Pethidine.

The order must contain the following:

- Name of the midwife
- Occupation of the midwife
- Name of the person to whom the Controlled Drug is to be administered or supplied
- Purpose for which the Controlled Drug is required
- Total quantity of the drug to be obtained
- Signature of an appropriate medical officer – a doctor authorised (in writing) by the local supervising authority or the person appointed by the supervising authority to exercise supervision over midwives within the area.

For details on checking registration of nurses see section 3.3.16.

3.7.7 PRESCRIPTION REQUIREMENTS FOR SCHEDULE 2 AND 3 CONTROLLED DRUGS

The requirements that must be present for a prescription (both NHS and private) for Schedule 2 or 3 Controlled Drugs to be valid are outlined in Diagram 14 (see section 3.3.1 for the usual prescription requirements which also apply). For private prescriptions see also Table 15 for information on the standardised forms that must be used.

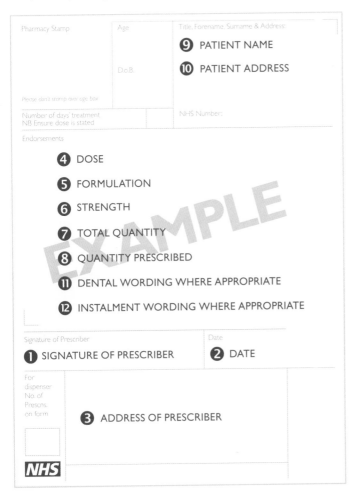

DIAGRAM 14: CONTROLLED DRUG PRESCRIPTION REQUIREMENTS FOR SCHEDULE 2 OR 3 CONTROLLED DRUGS

❶ **SIGNATURE** – the prescription needs to be signed by the prescriber with their usual signature. The pharmacist should either recognise the signature (and believe it to be genuine) or take reasonable steps to satisfy themselves that it is genuine. The prescription may be signed by another prescriber other than the named prescriber and still be legally valid. However, the address of the prescriber needs to be applicable to the signatory for the prescription to be legally compliant. The Controlled Drugs register entry should record the details of the actual prescriber (the signatory) rather than the named prescriber. Doctors, dentists, vets, supplementary nurse or pharmacist prescribers (subject to a clinical management plan), independent nurse prescribers and pharmacist independent prescribers can prescribe Controlled Drugs. Advanced electronic signatures can be accepted for Schedule 2 and 3 Controlled Drugs where the Electronic Prescribing Service (EPS) is used.

❷ **DATE** – the prescription needs to include the date on which it was signed. Controlled drugs prescriptions are valid for 28 days after the appropriate date on the prescription. The appropriate date is either the signature date or any other date indicated on the prescription (by the prescriber) as a date before which the drugs should not be supplied – whichever is later. The 28 day restriction includes prescriptions for Schedule 4 Controlled Drugs and any owing balances (see section 3.3.1 for details on the validity of owings).

③ PRESCRIBER'S ADDRESS – the address of the prescriber must be included on the prescription and must be within the UK.

④ DOSE – the dose does not need to be in both words and figures; however, it must be clearly defined (see Table 14).

⑤ FORMULATION – the formulation must be stated; the abbreviations 'tabs' and 'caps' are acceptable.

⑥ STRENGTH – the strength only needs to be written on the prescription if the medicine is available in more than one strength. To avoid ambiguity, where a prescription requests multiple strengths of a medicine, each strength should be prescribed separately (i.e. separate dose, total quantity, etc.).

⑦ TOTAL QUANTITY – the total quantity must be written in both words and figures. If the medicine is in dosage units (tablets, capsules, ampoules, millilitres, etc), the Home Office advises this should be expressed as a number of dosage units (e.g. 10 tablets [of 10mg] rather than 100mg total quantity). The total quantity can be expressed as the multiplication of two numbers provided both components are clearly and unambiguously written in words and figures (e.g. '2 packs of 30 tablets; two packs of thirty tablets'. Liquids should be expressed as millilitres. (For information on amendments pharmacists can make see 'Technical errors').

⑧ QUANTITY PRESCRIBED – the Department of Health and the Scottish Government have issued strong recommendations that the maximum quantity of Schedule 2, 3 or 4 Controlled Drugs prescribed should not exceed 30 days. This is not a legal restriction but prescribers should be able to justify the quantity requested (on a clinical basis) if more than 30 days' supply is prescribed. There may be genuine circumstances for which medicines need to be prescribed in this way.

⑨ NAME OF PATIENT

⑩ ADDRESS OF PATIENT – if the patient does not have a fixed address (e.g. because he or she is homeless or under a witness protection scheme), 'no fixed abode' or 'NFA' is acceptable. Use of a PO Box is not acceptable.

⑪ DENTAL PRESCRIPTIONS – where the Controlled Drug prescription is written by a dentist, the words 'for dental treatment only' must be present.

⑫ INSTALMENT DIRECTION – where the prescription is intended to be supplied in instalments a valid instalment direction is required. (For further information see 'Instalment direction for Schedule 2 or 3 Controlled Drugs').

Additional requirements: When the Controlled Drug is supplied, it is a requirement to mark the prescription with the date of supply at the time the supply is made. The prescription needs to be written in indelible ink and can be computer generated.

Sugar free products: Pharmacists are reminded that sugar free and/or colour free products have a greater potential for abuse; therefore the RPS advise that these are only supplied when specifically prescribed.

Name of the medicine

Clearly, the name of the prescribed medicine is necessary on a prescription to identify which medicine is being requested. However, it is not a legal requirement. It is good practice to write the name of the medicine in full as it appears in the manufacturer's summary of product characteristics.

TABLE 14: EXAMPLES OF DOSES THAT ARE, AND ARE NOT, LEGALLY ACCEPTABLE (NOT EXHAUSTIVE)

EXAMPLES OF DOSES THAT ARE NOT LEGALLY ACCEPTABLE	EXAMPLES OF DOSES THAT ARE LEGALLY ACCEPTABLE (*NB: LEGAL ACCEPTABILITY DOES NOT AUTOMATICALLY INDICATE CLINICAL APPROPRIATENESS*)
As directed	One as directed
When required	Two when required
PRN	One PRN
As per chart	Three ampoules to be given as directed (better still – three ampoules to be given over 24 hours as directed)
Titration dose	
Weekly (this is just a frequency and not a dose)	
Decrease dose by 3.5ml every four days	One to two when required

Instalment direction for Schedule 2 or 3 Controlled Drugs

An instalment direction combines two pieces of information:

1. Amount of medicine per instalment.
2. Interval between each time the medicine can be supplied.

The Home Office has confirmed that an instalment prescription must have both a dose and an instalment amount specified separately on the prescription.

The first instalment must be dispensed within 28 days of the appropriate date (see *Date* Diagram 14). The remainder of the instalments should be dispensed in accordance with the instructions (even if this runs beyond 28 days after the appropriate date).

NEW HOME OFFICE APPROVED WORDING FOR INSTALMENT PRESCRIBING

The Home Office introduced a new set of approved wording for instalment prescribing in November 2015. This new set of wording is shorter in length and more flexible than the previous set of approved wording. The expectation is that prescribers will take steps to move from using the old approved wording to the new set of approved wording in the coming months.

The Home Office recognise that it will take time for the introduction of the new wording to be implemented and so all legal prescriptions which incorporate the old wording clearly establishing the intentions of the prescriber should continue to be accepted and dispensed as is currently the case, unless in the professional judgment of the pharmacist there are reasons why these prescriptions should not be accepted. Prescribers must use either the new wording or the old wording but not a combination of both or an amended version of the old wording. The old wording can be found for reference purposes on the RPS website (**www.rpharms.com/support/mep.asp**).

If the only date on the prescription is the date of signing, the first dispensing needs to take place within 28 days of this date. If the prescriber indicates on the prescription a date before which the prescribed medicine should not be dispensed, this would be the appropriate date instead. The prescription must then be marked with the date of each supply.

The instalment direction is a legal requirement and needs to be complied with. However, because there are acknowledged practical difficulties with missed doses and dates when the pharmacy is closed (e.g. bank holidays), the Home Office has approved specific wording to be used that gives pharmacists a degree of flexibility when making a supply.

The following wording allows a pharmacy to supply the balance of an instalment if the interval date is missed (i.e. if three days' supply was directed to be supplied on day 1 but it was missed, it allows two days' supply to be issued on day 2).

NEW SET OF APPROVED WORDING

1. Please dispense instalments due on pharmacy closed days on a prior suitable day.
2. If an instalment's collection day has been missed, please still dispense the amount due for any remaining day(s) of that instalment.
3. Consult the prescriber if 3 or more consecutive days of a prescription have been missed.
4. Supervise consumption on collection days.
5. Dispense daily doses in separate containers.

NB: If the prescriber selects instalment intervals that take bank holidays or other closure dates into account, it may not be necessary to include this wording.

NB: If you decide to supply against a prescription that uses wording not approved by the Home Office, it will not provide the same protection from enforcement when making the supply. In this instance, if practical, you should try to get the prescription amended by the prescriber to include the approved Home Office wording.

Missed doses

If you know a patient has missed three days' prescribed treatment (or the number of days defined by any local agreement with the prescriber), there is a risk that he or she will have lost tolerance to the drug and the usual dose may cause overdose. In the best interests of the patient, consider contacting the prescriber to discuss appropriate next steps.

Technical errors

Where a prescription for a Schedule 2 or 3 Controlled Drug contains a minor typographical error or spelling mistake, or where either the words or figures (but not both) of the total quantity has been omitted, a pharmacist can amend the prescription indelibly so that it becomes compliant with legislation.

The pharmacist needs to have exercised due diligence, be satisfied that the prescription is genuine and that the supply is in accordance with the intention of the prescriber. The prescription should also be marked to show that the amendments are attributable to the pharmacist (e.g. name, date, signature and GPhC registration number).

Pharmacists cannot correct other amendments or omissions (e.g. missing date, incorrect dose, form or strength). These should be corrected by the original prescriber or, in an emergency, another prescriber authorised to prescribe Controlled Drugs. Amendments cannot be made by covering letter from the prescriber.

Only medical prescribers who hold a special licence from the Home Secretary or Scottish Government's Chief Medical Officer can prescribe cocaine, diamorphine or dipipanone for treating addiction. This special licence is not required if treating organic disease or injury. Pharmacist independent prescribers, nurse independent prescribers and supplementary prescribers may not prescribe cocaine, diamorphine or dipipanone for treating addiction, but may prescribe these medicines for treating organic disease or injury.

The handling of Controlled Drugs in prisons requires specific processes underpinned by the information currently found in the NPC document (UK Web Archive) *Safe Management and Use of Controlled Drugs in Prison Health in England* **(www.webarchive.org.uk/wayback/archive/20140627111322/http://www.npc.nhs.uk/controlled_drugs/).**

Private prescription requirements for Schedule 2 and 3 Controlled Drugs

1. STANDARDISED FORM

Following from the recommendations of the Shipman Inquiry, private prescriptions for Schedule 2 or 3 Controlled Drugs must be written on designated standardised forms. The forms that should be used are described in Table 15.

Private prescriptions that are not on the designated standardised form must not be accepted unless they are veterinary prescriptions.

For a hospital pharmacy to lawfully supply a Schedule 2 or 3 Controlled Drug against a private prescription issued outside that hospital (i.e. outside its legal entity), a standardised form must be used. Where the private prescription is issued and dispensed within the same legal entity, a standardised form is not required.

TABLE 15: CONTROLLED DRUGS PRIVATE PRESCRIPTION FORMS

	ENGLAND	SCOTLAND	WALES
FORM THAT MUST BE USED	FP10CD	PPCD(1)	WP10PCD
WHERE TO OBTAIN FORMS	Local NHS England area team	Local NHS health board	Local NHS health board

2. PRESCRIBER IDENTIFICATION NUMBER

A prescriber identification number must be included on standardised private prescriptions. This number is not the prescriber's professional registration number (i.e. the GMC number). It is a number issued by the relevant NHS agency and the prescriber can obtain it from their local primary care organisation. In Scotland, a valid NHS prescriber code is used where available or new ones issued where necessary.

3. SUBMISSION

Pharmacies must submit the original private prescription to the relevant NHS agency (NHS Business Services Authority or equivalent); for veterinary prescriptions see below. This requires an identifying code assigned to the pharmacy for this purpose by the local primary care organisation.

VETERINARY PRESCRIPTIONS

Veterinary prescriptions for Controlled Drugs do not need to be written on standardised forms nor do they need to be submitted to the relevant NHS agency. Forms must be retained for five years.

The Veterinary Pharmacists Group virtual network is available to members on the RPS website (www.rpharms.com).

PRACTICE ISSUES: PRESCRIBING OTHER MEDICINES ON THE SAME FORM AS CONTROLLED DRUGS

Medicines that are not Controlled Drugs should not be prescribed on the same form as a Schedule 2 or 3 Controlled Drug. This is because the form needs to be sent to the relevant NHS agency so the pharmacist would be unable to comply with the requirement to keep private prescriptions for a POM for two years.

FURTHER READING

NHS Business Services Authority. *Private CD prescribers.* **(www.nhsbsa.nhs.uk/ PrescriptionServices/3993.aspx)**

Information Services Division Scotland. *Private prescribers of Controlled Drugs.* **(www.isdscotland. org/Health-Topics/Prescribing-and-Medicines/ Prescriber-Codes)**

3.7.8 COLLECTION OF DISPENSED CONTROLLED DRUGS

When a Schedule 2 Controlled Drug is collected from a pharmacy, the pharmacist is legally required to determine whether the person collecting is a patient, patient's representative or healthcare professional.

Depending upon which type of person is collecting, the pharmacist needs to take appropriate action (see Table 16). See also section 3.7.11 for further information on record keeping requirements.

TABLE 16: ACTIONS REQUIRED WHEN A DISPENSED SCHEDULE 2 CONTROLLED DRUG IS COLLECTED

PERSON COLLECTING	ACTION	NOTES
PATIENT	Pharmacist may request evidence of that person's identity, unless already known to the pharmacist	The decision whether to supply or not is at the discretion of the supplying pharmacist – based on their professional judgement
PATIENT'S REPRESENTATIVE		
*HEALTHCARE PROFESSIONAL ACTING IN THEIR PROFESSIONAL CAPACITY ON BEHALF OF THE PATIENT	Unless already known to the pharmacist, obtain: 1. Name of healthcare professional 2. Address of healthcare professional Also request evidence of identity	Where evidence of identity is not available, the pharmacist has discretion over whether to supply or not – based on their professional judgement

*In this scenario, 'healthcare professional' refers to any person authorised to collect a Schedule 2 Controlled Drug medication on behalf of the person named on the prescription who is operating under a contract of employment in a health or social care occupation (for example a doctor, nurse or care worker)

Collection by a representative of a drug misuse patient

If a drug misuser wants a representative to collect a dispensed Controlled Drug on his or her behalf, pharmacists are advised to first obtain a letter from the drug misuser that authorises and names the representative. (This includes those detained in police custody who should supply a letter of authorisation to a police custody officer to present to the pharmacist). A separate letter should be obtained each time the drug misuser sends a representative to collect and the representative should bring identification. The pharmacist must be satisfied that the letter is genuine. It is also good practice to insist on seeing the patient in person at least once a week unless this is known not to be possible. The record of supply in the Controlled Drug register should include details of the representative.

If the directions on the prescription state that the dose must be supervised, the pharmacist should contact the prescriber before the medicine is supplied to the representative – since supervision will not be possible. It is legally acceptable to confirm verbally with the prescriber that they are happy with this arrangement since supervision, while important, is not a legal requirement under the 2001 Regulations. An appropriate record of this conversation should be made. It would not be necessary to contact the prescriber if the person has been detained in police custody and the representative collecting the dose is a police custody officer or a custody healthcare professional. This is because the administration of any Schedule 2 or 3 Controlled Drug in custody will be supervised by a healthcare professional. If the dose is usually supervised, but has been supplied, the pharmacist should consider annotating the prescription and patient medication records to advise others that the dose has not been supervised in the pharmacy.

PRACTICE ISSUES

- It is good practice for the person collecting a Schedule 2 or 3 Controlled Drug to sign the space on the reverse of the prescription form that is specifically for this purpose. A supply can be made if this is not signed, subject to the professional judgement of the pharmacist

- Instalment prescriptions only need to be signed once

- A representative, including a delivery driver, can sign on behalf of a patient. However, a robust audit trail should be available to confirm successful delivery of the medicine to the patient.

FURTHER READING

Public Health England. *Access to supervised doses of opioid substitution for people in police custody.* September 2015. (**http://www.nta.nhs.uk/prison-based.aspx**)

The concept of safe custody is derived from the Safe Custody Regulations and refers to the physical security of certain Schedule 2 or 3 Controlled Drugs. It requires that pharmacies, private hospitals and care homes keep relevant Controlled Drugs in a 'locked safe, cabinet or room which is constructed as to prevent unauthorised access to the drugs'. For settings other than those listed above, these regulations are considered minimum standards for safe custody.

Structural requirements of safes, cabinets and rooms used for storing Controlled Drugs

The structural requirements and technical details with which Controlled Drug safes, cabinets and rooms must comply are detailed in Schedule 2 of the Safe Custody Regulations. These requirements are of a technical nature requiring expertise and knowledge of construction. The Royal Pharmaceutical Society does not endorse or approve individual (or brands of) Controlled Drugs cabinets.

When purchasing a safe or cabinet, reassurance should be sought from the vendor or manufacturer that the product specifications comply with the requirements specified in the Safe Custody Regulations.

Alternatively, you must apply for an exemption certificate from the police, which certifies that the safe, cabinet or room provides an adequate degree of security for holding Controlled Drugs. For further information, contact your local police station.

The Controlled Drugs that must be kept under safe custody are:

- Schedule 1 drugs
- Schedule 2 drugs except some liquid preparations and quinalbarbitone (secobarbital). Details of exempted Schedule 2 Controlled Drugs are available from the Misuse of Drugs (Safe Custody) Regulations 1973 as amended
- Schedule 3 drugs unless exempted under the Misuse of Drugs (Safe Custody) Regulations 1973 as amended, where the full lists are available. Common exemptions include: phenobarbital, mazindol, meprobamate, midazolam, tramadol, pentazocine and phentermine

- Common Schedule 3 Controlled Drugs which require safe custody include temazepam and buprenorphine.

SAFE CUSTODY REQUIREMENTS FOR SECURE ENVIRONMENTS AND SECONDARY CARE

Prison building regulations specify details of the robust nature required for all rooms that store Controlled Drugs. For further information, see the Ministry of Justice's PSI 45/2010 Prison Service Order for Integrated Drug Treatment System (www.justice.gov.uk)

In prisons and hospitals, it is recommended that the CD cabinet should meet the 'Sold Secure silver standard'. For further information, see:

- **National Prescribing Centre** (UK Web Archive). *A guide to good practice in the management of Controlled Drugs in primary care* (England). December 2009. (http://www.webarchive.org.uk/wayback/archive/20140627111322/http://www.npc.nhs.uk/controlled_drugs/)

- **Department of Health** (National Archives). *Safer management of Controlled Drugs: A guide to good practice in secondary care* (England). October 2007. (http://webarchive.nationalarchives.gov.uk/+/www.dh.gov.uk/en/Publicationsandstatistics/Publications/PublicationsPolicyAndGuidance/DH_074513)

- Health Building Notes 00-01 General design principles 14-01 Designing pharmacy and radiopharmacy facilities (www.gov.uk/government/collections/health-building-notes-core-elements)

- Welsh Health Building Notes 00-01 General design principles 14-01 Designing pharmacy and radiopharmacy facilities (www.wales.nhs.uk).

UNDERPINNING KNOWLEDGE – LEGISLATION AND PROFESSIONAL ISSUES

Some organisations may carry out a risk assessment which determines that Controlled Drugs in Schedules 3, 4 and 5 should be handled in the same way as Controlled Drugs in Schedule 2. This may result in Controlled Drugs other than those that require safe custody by law, being stored in the Controlled Drugs safe, cabinet or room. This should be included in the relevant policy documents and standard operating procedures.

When Controlled Drugs requiring safe custody are not kept in the Controlled Drugs cabinet, safe or room (e.g. during the dispensing process), they must be under the 'direct personal supervision' of a pharmacist.

Access to Controlled Drugs (including handling of 'CD keys') should be documented within a policy. The policy should prevent unauthorised access and be able to identify who has had access to Controlled Drugs (e.g. the electronic logs from a room or cabinet with electronic access or an audit trail for holders of the CD keys). In community pharmacies, it is common for the pharmacist to hold the CD keys.

A key log could be used to keep an audit trail of who has had access to the keys, including overnight storage in the pharmacy, the transfer of the keys from one pharmacist at the end of a shift to another pharmacist,

etc. A template CD key log is available in the quick reference guide *Safe custody of Controlled Drugs* (http://rpharms.com/support-resources/support-resources-a-z.asp)

Patient-returned and out-of-date or obsolete Controlled Drugs

Safe custody applies to patient-returned, out-of-date and obsolete Controlled Drugs until they can be destroyed (see section 3.7.10). To minimise the risk of supplying these to patients, this stock should be segregated from other pharmacy stock and be clearly marked (e.g. mark the stock as 'patient returns waiting to be destroyed' or 'out of date, waiting authorised witness to destroy', etc).

FURTHER READING

RPS *quick reference guide. Safe custody of Controlled Drugs.*
(www.rpharms.com/resources-AtoZ)
Appelbe GE, Wingfield J, editors. *Dale and Applebe's Pharmacy and Medicines Law.* 10th edition. London: Pharmaceutical Press; 2013.

3.7.10 DESTRUCTION OF CONTROLLED DRUGS

Pharmacies are required to denature Controlled Drugs prior to disposal. Usually, this process requires an appropriate licence but pharmacies are exempt from needing one (although they must register their exemption). Registration of an exemption is different from obtaining a licence.

In England and Wales, an exemption is issued by the Environment Agency and is known as the 'T28 exemption'. This allows pharmacies to sort and dispose of Controlled Drugs and to comply with the 2001 Regulations by denaturing them prior to disposal. This exemption needs to be registered with the Environment Agency, which can be done on their website (**www.gov.uk/government/organisations/environment-agency**).

In Scotland, the exemption is issued by the Scottish Environment Protection Agency (SEPA), which currently accepts that the denaturing of Controlled Drugs forms part of the exempt activity of secure storage.

Both the Environment Agency and SEPA have indicated that they may reconsider their positions at any time and may pursue enforcement action where activities cause, or are likely to cause, environmental pollution or harm to human health.

Controlled Drugs that need to be denatured before disposal

The Home Office has advised that all Controlled Drugs in Schedules 2, 3 and 4 (part 1) should be denatured and, therefore, rendered irretrievable before disposal.

Persons authorised to witness the denaturing of Controlled Drugs

In some circumstances, the denaturing of Controlled Drugs needs to be witnessed by an authorised person. Where there is a requirement to make a Controlled Drug register entry, legislation also requires to have their destruction witnessed. Typically, the destruction of pharmacy stock of Schedule 2 Controlled Drugs needs to be witnessed. The destruction of patient-returned Controlled Drugs, whether they require denaturing or not, does not require witnessing by an authorised person.

Table 17 summarises the denaturing and witnessing requirements for patient-returned and expired Controlled Drugs.

TABLE 17: DENATURING AND WITNESS REQUIREMENTS FOR PATIENT-RETURNED AND EXPIRED CONTROLLED DRUGS

	IS DENATURING REQUIRED?	IS AN AUTHORISED WITNESS REQUIRED?	RECORD KEEPING
PATIENT-RETURNED CONTROLLED DRUG	Yes, if Schedule 2, 3 or 4 (part 1)	No. However it is preferable for denaturing to be witnessed by another member of staff familiar with Controlled Drugs (preferably a registered health professional)	A record should not be made in the Controlled Drugs register but records of patient-returned Schedule 2 Controlled Drugs and their subsequent destruction should be recorded in a separate record for this purpose
EXPIRED/OBSOLETE/ UNWANTED STOCK	Yes, if Schedule 2, 3 or 4 (part 1)	Yes, if Schedule 2. For Schedule 3 medicines it would be good practice to have another member of staff witness the denaturing	An entry should be made in the Controlled Drug register for Schedule 2 Controlled Drugs

NB: If a pharmacy is engaged in manufacturing, compounding, importing or exporting Schedule 3 or 4 Controlled Drugs then record keeping arrangements apply. Therefore, destruction of these requires an authorised witness.

In prisons, to maintain a robust audit trail, use of Schedule 3 Controlled Drugs (e.g. buprenorphine) should be recorded in the Controlled Drugs register. Therefore, any destruction should also be recorded. It is also recommended that a robust audit trail is maintained for Schedule 4 Controlled Drugs, such as diazepam and chlordiazepoxide.

Various individuals and classes of person (e.g. police constables) are authorised to witness the destruction of Controlled Drugs. This authority is derived from the Home Secretary. It can also be derived from the Secretary of State for Health or from an accountable officer (see section 3.7.1). An accountable officer has the power to authorise other persons to witness the destruction of Controlled Drugs. However the 2001 Regulations prevent an accountable officer from being an authorised person directly. Persons authorised by the accountable officer are usually senior members of staff who are not involved in the day-to-day management or use of Controlled Drugs.

Methods of denaturing Controlled Drugs

All medicines should be disposed of in a safe and appropriate manner. Medicines should be disposed of in appropriate waste containers that are then sent for incineration. They should not be disposed of into the sewerage system.

The following generic advice has been agreed with the Home Office.

All Controlled Drugs in Schedule 2, 3 and 4 (part 1) should be destroyed by being denatured and rendered irretrievable before being placed into pharmaceutical waste containers and sent for incineration.

The context of destruction by denaturing and rendering irretrievable is to guard against the misuse of drugs, harm to the environment or people and prevent the supply of easily retrievable Controlled Drugs to waste carriers. These methods are not expected to render the detection of active ingredients with specialist equipment impossible, or to modify the chemical composition or properties of CDs.

For all forms of denaturing, and particularly if grinding or crushing tablets or breaking containers is involved individuals should work in a well-ventilated area and wear suitable protective gloves, a face mask and goggles as appropriate; following good Health and Safety practice.

Table 18 contains generic advice on methods of denaturing which have been agreed with the Home Office as likely to be compatible with legislative requirements. If additional product specific information is needed speak to the manufacturer of the product or your local Controlled Drug accountable officer.

Controlled Drug denaturing kits designed specifically for this purpose are widely available and should be used in preference to other materials that were historically used such as cat litter. It is the responsibility of the manufacturer or supplier of the kit to ensure that the kit and the instructions for use are fit-for-purpose. Pharmacists are responsible for using a kit that has been obtained from a reputable source and to use those kits in accordance with the manufacturers' instructions – generic advice is also available in Table 18.

TABLE 18: DESTRUCTION OF CONTROLLED DRUGS

DOSAGE FORM	METHOD OF DESTRUCTION
SOLID DOSAGE FORMS, E.G. CAPSULES AND TABLETS	Grind or crush the solid dose formulation before adding to the CD denaturing kit to ensure that whole tablets or capsules are not retrievable. The use of a small amount of water whilst grinding or crushing may assist in minimising particles of dust being released into the air.
	Where a CD denaturing kit is not available, an alternative method of denaturing is to crush or grind the solid dose formulation and place it into a small amount of warm, soapy water stirring sufficiently to ensure the drug has been dissolved or dispersed. The resulting mixture may then be poured onto an appropriate amount of suitable product* and added to an appropriate waste disposal bin supplied by the waste contractor.
LIQUID DOSAGE FORMS	Pour into an appropriately sized CD denaturing kit.
	Where a CD denaturing kit is not available, an alternative method is to pour the liquid onto an appropriate amount of suitable product* and then to add this to an appropriate waste disposal bin.

DOSAGE FORM	METHOD OF DESTRUCTION
AMPOULES AND VIALS	For liquid containing ampoules, open the ampoule and empty the contents into a CD denaturing kit, or dispose of in the same manner as liquid dose formulations above. Dispose of the ampoule as sharps pharmaceutical waste.
	For powder containing ampoules, open the ampoule and add water to dissolve the powder inside. The resulting mixture can be poured into the CD denaturing kit and the ampoule disposed of as sharps pharmaceutical waste.
	An alternative but less preferable, disposal method is where the ampoules are crushed with a pestle inside an empty plastic container. Once broken, a small quantity of warm soapy water (for powder ampoules) or suitable product* (for liquid ampoules) is added. If these methods are used, care should be taken to ensure that the glass does not harm the person destroying the CD. The resulting liquid mixture should then be disposed of in a CD denaturing kit or in the bin that is used for disposal of liquid medicines.
PATCHES	Remove the backing and fold the patch over on itself. Place into a waste disposal bin or a CD denaturing kit.
AEROSOL FORMULATIONS	Expel into water and dispose of the resulting liquid in accordance with the guidance above on destroying liquid formulations.
	If this is not possible because of the nature of the formulation, expel into an absorbent material and dispose of this as pharmaceutical waste.
	Alternatively consider if it would be safe to open or to otherwise compromise the container to release the Controlled Drug safely. The resulting liquid mixture should then be disposed of in a CD denaturing kit and disposed of as pharmaceutical waste.

A risk assessment should be carried out to determine whether a product is suitable. A suitable product should render the Controlled Drug irretrievable without compromising patient safety, the safety of the person carrying out the destruction, or the environment.

3.7.11 RECORD KEEPING AND CONTROLLED DRUGS REGISTERS

A Controlled Drugs register must be used to record details of any Schedule 1 and Schedule 2 Controlled Drugs received or supplied by a pharmacy.

Pharmacists are also required to keep records of Sativex (which is a Schedule 4 Part 1 Controlled Drug). The Home Office strongly recommends the use of a Controlled Drug register for making records relating to Sativex.

For Controlled Drugs **received**, the following must be recorded:

- Date supply received
- Name and address from whom received
- Quantity received.

For Controlled Drugs **supplied**, the following must be recorded:

- Date supplied

- Name and address of recipient
- Details of authority to possess – prescriber or licence holder's details
- Quantity supplied
- Details of person collecting Schedule 2 Controlled Drug – patient, patient's representative or healthcare representative (if the latter, also record their name and address)
- Whether proof of identity was requested of the person collecting
- Whether proof of identity was provided.

These are the minimum fields of information that must be recorded; additional relevant information can be added without breaking the law.

THE NATURE OF THE REGISTER

Legislation requires that the class, strength and form be specified at the head of each page of the Controlled Drugs register. The register is required to be a bound book register (see box overleaf titled *Electronic Controlled Drugs register* for alternative to bound). It is also a requirement that different classes are kept in a separate part of the register and that, within each class, a separate page is used for different strengths and formulations of each drug. Multiple registers for the same class of Controlled Drug are allowable if approved by the Home Office.

Prisons have one legally compliant register that records all the details as specified. However, since there are often several areas in each prison where Controlled Drugs are stored, administered or issued, each of these areas should maintain a Controlled Drug record book (similar to those used by hospital wards). Also recommended is that the movement of Controlled Drugs between these areas be recorded by internal requisition so that robust audit trails are maintained.

THE NATURE OF THE ENTRIES

All entries made in Controlled Drugs registers should be:

■ **Entered chronologically**

■ **Entered promptly** – entries must be made on the day of the transaction or on the following day

■ **In ink or indelible** – entries and corrections must be in ink or indelible (or computerised [see below])

■ **Unaltered** – entries must not be cancelled, obliterated or altered. Corrections must be made by dated marginal notes or footnotes. The register should be marked to show who the amendments made are attributable to (e.g. name, initials/signature, GPhC number if applicable).

RECORD KEEPING

The following points regarding record keeping should be adhered to when maintaining Controlled Drugs registers:

■ **Location** – each register should be kept at the premises to which it applies

■ **Duration** – registers should be kept for two years from the date of the last entry

■ **Form** – records can be kept in their original form or copied and kept in an approved computerised form

■ **Inspection** – a copy of the register, and other details of stock, receipts and supplies, must be made available to authorised persons (e.g. a General Pharmaceutical Council inspector or Controlled Drug liaison officer) upon request.

ELECTRONIC CONTROLLED DRUGS REGISTERS

Electronic Controlled Drugs registers are permitted as an alternative to having a bound-book Controlled Drugs register. Legislation requires that computerised entries must be:

- Attributable
- Capable of being audited
- Compliant with best practice.

An electronic Controlled Drugs register must also be accessible from the premises and capable of being printed.

Registers may only be kept in computerised form if safeguards are incorporated into the software to ensure all of the following:

- The author of each entry is identifiable
- Entries cannot be altered at a later date
- A log of all data entered is kept and can be recalled for audit purposes.

Access control systems should be in place to minimise the risk of unauthorised or unnecessary access to the data. Adequate backups must be made of computerised registers. Arrangements should be made so that inspectors can examine computerised registers during a visit with minimum disruption to the dispensing process.

Running balances and stock checks

The aim of a running balance is to ensure that irregularities or discrepancies are identified as quickly as possible. A standard operating procedure (SOP) should be in place for stock checks of all Controlled Drugs that are recorded in the Controlled Drugs register. This should include checking the running balance in the register against the physical amount of stock, frequency of stock checks and details of how stock checks of liquids should be carried out. For most organisations the frequency of stock checks should be at least once a week* but these may be more or less frequent based on risk assessment, volume of Controlled Drugs dispensing, frequency of past irregularities or incidents, or if there are several different pharmacists in charge over short periods. Liquid balances should be checked visually with periodic volume checks, and checks to confirm the balance on completion of a bottle. Stock checks should be recorded, signed and dated by the healthcare professional carrying out the check and if possible, two people should carry out stock checks.

It is also appropriate to visually check the running balance each time a Controlled Drug is dispensed (i.e. where the calculated balance in the register visually matches the quantity you can see. If it does not match, you should investigate in more detail).

Some common reasons for stock to be at zero balance could be due to the drug not being reordered, destruction of the drug (i.e. expired and obsolete, see section 3.7.10 for destruction of Controlled Drugs) or discontinuation of the drug by the manufacturer. Pharmacists can exercise their professional judgement to help decide whether the weekly running balance check for these Controlled Drug(s) that have been zero balance for some time should be continued or suspended. Referring to relevant SOP(s) could form part of this process.

A running balance should be maintained as a matter of good practice and is a recommendation from the Shipman Inquiry. (It is intended that once electronic registers are in common use this will become a legal requirement).

Once a week, not necessarily required to be on the same day every week.

- The pharmacist has overall responsibility for maintaining running balances and dealing with discrepancies. However, these tasks can be delegated to competent staff, where appropriate

- If a discrepancy can be resolved following checks, a marginal note or footnote should be made in the register and the discrepancy corrected

- An SOP should be written for how to check running balances and deal with discrepancies. This SOP should include instructions for when the owner or superintendent, GPhC inspector, accountable officer or Controlled Drug liaison officer should be notified of discrepancies

- Running balances for liquid Controlled Drugs can be affected by overage, residue and spillage

- Where a CD register entry has been made for a Schedule 2 Controlled Drug, the usual requirement to make a record in the POM register does not apply.

3.7.12 PRACTICE ISSUES: DISPOSING OF SPENT METHADONE BOTTLES

NICE has published guidance on the disposal of stock Controlled Drugs bottles that contain irretrievable amounts of liquid drugs. Once the stock bottle has been emptied as far as possible (within the dispensing process), bottles should be rinsed and the liquid disposed of into a pharmaceutical waste bin. Disposal of irretrievable amounts of controlled drugs does not need to be recorded. For patient returned liquid Controlled Drug containers, any excess liquid must be denatured. The container should then be rinsed out and the rinsing added to the denaturing kit. For both stock and patient returned containers, labels and other identifiers should be removed or obliterated and the clean, empty container disposed of into the recycling or general waste.

FURTHER READING

Department of Health. *Safe management of healthcare waste* 2013. (**www.gov.uk/government/publications/guidance-on-the-safe-management-of-healthcare-waste**)

NICE. *Controlled drugs: safe use and management.* April 2016. (**www.nice.org.uk**)

UNDERPINNING KNOWLEDGE – LEGISLATION AND PROFESSIONAL ISSUES

3.7.13 PRACTICE ISSUES: NEEDLE EXCHANGE SCHEME

Pharmacists who are delivering or contemplating on providing a needle exchange service should be aware of national guidelines:

England and Wales – *NICE public health guidance 52. Needle and syringe programmes.* March 2014. **(www.nice.org.uk)**

Scotland – *National guidelines for services providing injecting equipment.* 2010. **(www.gov.scot/Publications/2010/03/29165055/0)**

3.7.14 EXTEMPORANEOUS METHADONE

The GPhC has published guidance on the preparation of unlicensed medicines, which sets out the key areas that need to be considered by the pharmacy owner and superintendent pharmacist in any registered pharmacy where unlicensed medicines are prepared by a pharmacist or under the supervision of a pharmacist. Every patient has every right to expect that when an unlicensed medicine is prepared by, or under the supervision of, a registered pharmacist in a registered pharmacy, it is of equivalent quality to a licensed medicine.

This guidance also applies when unlicensed methadone is extemporaneously prepared. The guidance explains that pharmacies preparing unlicensed medicines, including the extemporaneous preparation of methadone, must mitigate risks to patients and meet the GPhC's standards for registered pharmacies.

The guidance was published in May 2014.

FURTHER RESOURCES
GPhC. *Standards for registered pharmacies* **see Appendix 2** or **www.pharmacyregulation.org** **GPhC.** *Guidance for registered pharmacies preparing unlicensed medicines* **see Appendix 12** or **www.pharmacyregulation.org**

4. ROYAL PHARMACEUTICAL SOCIETY RESOURCES

The following resources are available from our website (**www.rpharms.com**):

Pharmacy law and ethics

- Controlled Drugs
- Controlled Drugs: requisition requirements
- Dispensing and preparing extemporaneous methadone
- Drugs and driving
- EEA prescriptions
- Emergency supply
- Independent prescribing of Controlled Drugs
- Medicines, Ethics and Practice: The professional guide for pharmacists
- Poisons and chemicals from a pharmacy
- Professional judgement
- Professional support bulletins (RPS website)
- Pseudoephedrine and ephedrine
- Responsible Pharmacist hub
- Safe custody of Controlled Drugs
- Supply of medicines to podiatrists and their patients
- Veterinary medicines.

Reclassified medicines

- Amorolfine nail lacquer
- Azithromycin
- Chloramphenicol eye drops and eye ointment
- Omeprazole
- Oral emergency contraceptives as pharmacy medicines
- Orlistat
- Sumatriptan
- Tamsulosin
- Tranexamic acid P medicine.

Pharmacy practice

- 8 Core principles for community pharmacy whistle blowing policies and procedures
- Advertising pharmacy services and medication
- Best practice for ensuring the efficient supply and distribution of medicines to patients
- Care homes: Safety of medicines in care homes framework
- Children collecting medicines from a pharmacy
- Cholesterol testing
- Clinical governance
- Community pharmacy reforms
- Cough and cold products for children
- Dispensing oral isotretinoin and pregnancy prevention
- Dispensing valproate for girls and women
- Electronic Health Records (EHR)
- Essential Guide to Community Pharmacy Practice: Preparing for Day 1
- Explaining Biosimilar Medicines
- Flu: setting up a flu vaccination service via patient group direction
- Good dispensing guidelines – England
- GPhC premises standards and inspection report
- Handling of medicines in social care
- Homeopathic and herbal products
- Ibuprofen, isopropyl myristate topical P medicine
- Identification of foreign medicines
- Improving patient outcomes through better use of multi-compartment compliance aids (MCA)
- Locum pharmacists: Working as a locum pharmacist in community
- Managing medicines shortages in secondary care (England)

- Medical devices
- Medicines administration (MAR) charts: Principles of safe and appropriate production
- Medicines optimisation
- Medicines that optometrists can order
- Monitoring blood pressure
- Near miss error log
- NHS community pharmacy contract (England)
- NHS community pharmacy contract (Wales)
- Nurses, pharmacists and patient pathways: Working together across primary and community care
- Optimising dispensing labels and medicines use
- Oral emergency contraceptives as pharmacy medicines
- Pharmaceutical services to social care settings
- Pharmacy and the Olympics
- Protecting children and young people
- Protecting vulnerable adults
- Raising concerns, whistle blowing and speaking up safely in pharmacy
- Repeat medication management, prescription collection and delivery service
- Safe and effective use of medicines; Risk minimisation activities
- Safe and secure handling of medicines (Revised Duthie Report)
- Social media
- Specials
- Summary care records
- Supply of salbutamol inhalers to schools
- The right culture
- The traditional herbal medicine registration scheme
- Use of Welsh language in pharmacy.

Online Hub Pages

- Community pharmacy hub
- Hospital pharmacy hub
- Patient engagement hub
- Responsible Pharmacist
- The ultimate guide for pharmacist working in care homes (coming soon)
- The ultimate guide for pharmacists working in GP practices
- The ultimate guide for pharmacists working in urgent and emergency care (coming soon).

Clinical aspects of pharmacy

- Asthma: Medicines optimisation briefing
- Bowel cancer
- Cardiovascular: Medicines optimisation briefing
- Clinical check
- Counselling patients on medicines
- Diabetes
- Diagnostic testing and screening services
- Dispensing and supply of oral chemotherapy and systemic anticancer medicines in primary care
- How to use the BNF
- How to use the BNFC
- Improving practice and reducing risk in the provision of parental nutrition for neonates and children
- Lung cancer
- Medication adherence
- Medication history
- Medication review
- Oesophago-gastric cancer
- Ovarian cancer
- Supporting patients on oral anticoagulants
- Supporting patients with asthma
- Supporting patients with chronic obstructing pulmonary disease (COPD).

Public health issues

- Alcohol use disorders
- Dementia: Pharmacy and the call to action
- Ebola
- Mental health
- Mental health toolkit
- Obesity and weight management
- Seasonal influenza
- Sexual health
- Smoking cessation.

Professional standards

- Homecare Services
- Hospital pharmacy
- Interim statement of professional standard – supply of over the counter (OTC) medicines
- Public Health
- Referral Toolkit
- Transfer of Care.

Resources for professional development

- Faculty
- Foundation
- You and your career
  - Student resources
  - Pre-registration trainees
  - Recently qualified pharmacists
- Developing your practice
  - Developing leadership
  - Leadership framework
  - Pharmacist prescribers

- Careers support
  - Return to practice
- CPD
- Mentoring
- Workforce and education
- Tutors
- Expert advisory panels
- Qualified Persons.

Science and research

- Clinical audits
- Map of evidence
- New medicines, better medicines, better use of medicines
- Pharmaceutical science
- Research funding
- Research ready
- Research support and guidance
- Science and research education.

Other resources

- E-Alerts and RPS professional support updates
- E-Library (RPS electronic library for access to books and full text journal databases)
- Essential websites for pharmacists.

5. PROFESSIONAL STANDARDS

The RPS provides professional standards which are developed and owned by the profession that describe good practice, systems of care or working. Professional standards are supportive and enabling whilst also professionally challenging, describing and building on good practice to support pharmacists to achieve excellence in professional practice. They provide a broad framework to support pharmacists and their teams to develop their professional practice, improve services, shape future services and deliver high quality patient care across all settings and sectors. The professional standards can be used in different ways by pharmacists, and their teams, working in a variety of settings and roles. Professional standards support pharmacists and their teams as part of the continuous process of professional development supporting them with their journey to excellence.

The GPhC and RPS published a joint statement *Using standards and guidance to ensure patient centred professionalism in the delivery of care* in July 2014. This aims to highlight the importance of regulatory and professional standards and guidance as a way to protect patient safety and to promote responsibility and professionalism.

The joint statement explains that regulatory and professional standards have the same overarching purpose, to provide a framework that helps to ensure good care which is focused on patients.

The statement makes clear that pharmacists should always consider what is in the best interests of the patient. It also states that pharmacy professionals must be guided by their education and training and ongoing CPD, consider the standards and guidance (both regulatory and professional) that are relevant to the situation, and understand the legal framework in which they are operating.

The joint statement can be viewed on the RPS website at: **http://www.rpharms.com/what-s-happening-/news_show.asp?id=1249.asp** or on the GPhC website at: **www.pharmacyregulation.org**

Professional bodies and royal colleges are widely accepted by the healthcare and regulatory system as having a critical role and valuable insight in supporting healthcare professionals in their pursuit of delivering high quality care through professional standards and guidance on professional practice[1, 2].

The RPS has created the following professional standards and guidance principles:

- Professional standards for Hospital Pharmacy Services
- Interim statement of professional standard for the Supply of OTC Medicines
- Public Health standards for pharmacy
- Transfer of Care principles
- Medicines Optimisation principles (England)
- Homecare Services.

1. Quality in the new Health System – Maintaining and improving quality from April 2013 **www.gov.uk**
2. GPhC Standards of conduct, ethics and performance – standard 6.6. **www.pharmacyregulation.org**

PROFESSIONAL STANDARDS FOR HOSPITAL PHARMACY SERVICES

We published *Professional Standards for Hospital Pharmacy Services: Optimising patient outcomes from medicines* in July 2012. These ten overarching standards which have been developed by a wide range of stakeholders cover pharmacy services delivered by acute, mental health, private and community service providers. The standards aim to ensure that patients receive a high quality pharmacy service, from admission through to discharge across multiple care pathways, and underpin the patient experience and the safe, effective management of medicines within and across organisations.

In addition to the standards, a range of supporting resources including a handbook have been published.

In 2014, we re-launched the refreshed professional standards, which were revisited in light of the Francis Review of events at Mid Staffordshire Foundation Trust and the response to that review, the report of the National Advisory Group on the Safety of Patients in England (commonly referred to as the Berwick Report). More emphasis was given to some key themes such as increasing patient involvement and feedback and organisational culture. The standards were also reviewed to ensure they aligned with other developments in pharmacy and healthcare agendas in Scotland and Wales and we also incorporated the experience of the 35 development sites from across GB that spent a year putting the standards into practice. A summary of the changes to the standards is also available.

The *Professional Standards for Hospital Pharmacy Services* together with the development site report, seven day services for hospital pharmacy report, working together to help patients make the most of medicines report, the report on measuring patient experiences and supporting resources can be viewed on the RPS website at: **www.rpharms.com/unsecure-support-resources/professional-standards-for-hospital-pharmacy.asp**

INTERIM STATEMENT OF PROFESSIONAL STANDARD FOR THE SUPPLY OF OTC MEDICINES

In response to requests for professional guidance to support the supply of OTC medicines we created an interim standard in 2013. This has taken into account relevant pre-existing professional guidance, standards and RPS policy and provides additional context to minimum GPhC regulatory standards for registered pharmacies in the supply of OTC medicines.

The interim statement is available from the RPS website: **www.rpharms.com/unsecure-support-resources/interim-statement-of-professional-standard-supply-of-otc-medicines.asp**

PUBLIC HEALTH PRACTICE STANDARDS FOR PHARMACY

The *Professional Standards for Public Health Practice for Pharmacy* was published in 2014. This was developed by a group, led by the Royal Pharmaceutical Society, chaired by the Chief Executive, with input from pharmacy practitioners and experts in both pharmacy and public health from across Great Britain. Colleagues from the Department of Health, the Royal Society for Public Health (RSPH) and the Faculty of Public Health (FPH) joined pharmacists on this group.

The nine overarching standards are intended to provide a framework to help pharmacy teams, commissioners and those contracting services to design, implement, deliver and monitor high quality public health practice through pharmacy, regardless of the pharmacy settings from which services are delivered. The standards are also applicable to all levels of the pharmacy workforce across all settings, e.g. those working at specialist or strategic level, those working as a practitioner and the wider pharmacy workforce.

The standards align with existing resources and tools for the wider healthcare workforce, therefore, mirroring the nine core competency areas identified by the Faculty of Public Health (FPH). Aligning the professional standards for pharmacy with the FPH core areas supports pharmacy practitioners in delivering public health practice that is demonstrably consistent with other healthcare practitioners delivering public health.

The *Professional Standards for Public Health Practice for Pharmacy* have been developed to have wide appeal as they broadly align with pharmacy and public health developments in England and Wales. It is envisaged that elements of these standards will prove to be helpful as the RPS supports the Scottish Government in producing standards and guidance for pharmacists working in the NHS in Scotland.

The *Professional Standards for Public Health Practice for Pharmacy* and supporting resources can be viewed on the RPS website at: **www.rpharms.com/unsecure-support-resources/professional-standards-for-public-health.asp**

MEDICINES OPTIMISATION PRINCIPLES (ENGLAND)

Medicines remain the most common therapeutic intervention in healthcare. In May 2013 we published principles of 'medicines optimisation' as good practice guidance for health professionals in England to help patients to make the most of their medicines. These principles support the understanding of the patient's experience, evidence based choice of medicines, ensuring medicines use is as safe as possible and making medicines optimisation part of routine practice. The principles apply whether prescribing, dispensing, administering or taking medicines and are available from our website: **www.rpharms.com/what-we-re-working-on/medicines-optimisation.asp**

TRANSFER OF CARE PRINCIPLES

In July 2011 we published good practice guidance in the form of core principles for healthcare professionals and organisations to help keep patients safe when transferring between care providers. These resources are available from our website: **www.rpharms.com/previous-projects/getting-the-medicines-right.asp**

HOMECARE SERVICES

We published the *Professional Standards for Homecare Services* in 2013.

These overarching developmental standards give a broad framework which will support teams providing and commissioning homecare services to improve services continually and to shape future services and pharmacy roles to deliver quality patient care. These standards will help patients experience a consistent quality of homecare services, irrespective of homecare provider, that will protect them from incidents of avoidable harm and help them to get the best outcomes from their medicines.

In 2011 the Department of Health commissioned the report *Homecare Medicines – Towards a Vision for the Future*. The report made a list of recommendations to improve the financial and clinical governance arrangements for patients receiving medicines via the homecare route. In 2012, the Department of Health established a steering board chaired by the report's author, Mark Hackett, to oversee the implementation of the recommendations with a range of work streams including development of a framework of standards for homecare medicines. The *Professional Standards for Homecare Services,* developed by the Homecare Standards Workgroup, overseen by the Department of Health Homecare Strategy Board, and hosted and published by the RPS closely reflect the RPS *Professional Standards for Hospital Pharmacy Services*, and aim to ensure that patients receive safe, effective care from homecare services.

In May 2014 we published The Handbook for Homecare Services in England. This identifies currently available resources and good practice examples which may be used by homecare teams in the development of robust arrangements for compliance with the three domains of the Standard. Each section of the handbook contains information and guidance and signposts and identifies key documents that will help homecare teams manage homecare services within a clinical and financial governance framework as set out in the RPS standards. The Handbook for Homecare Services has been produced in parallel with the other 'Hackett' work streams to ensure consistency. Where appropriate the outputs of the other work streams are included in this handbook, or signposted from this handbook.

In September 2014 the Handbook for Homecare Services in Wales was published. The handbook has been adapted from the Handbook for Homecare Services in England with the support of the All Wales Medicines Homecare Committee and RPS Wales for use in NHS Wales to support organisations involved in the provision of medicines through homecare services in Wales to comply with the RPS standards and the key recommendations of the Hackett report.

The Homecare standards data collection form (self-assessment tool) can be used to record and evidence how the standards are implemented within your organisation.

The professional standards for homecare services and supporting resources can be viewed on the RPS website at: **www.rpharms.com/unsecure-support-resources/ professional-standards-for-homecare-services.asp**

6. ROYAL PHARMACEUTICAL SOCIETY CODE OF CONDUCT

The Code of Conduct for members of the Royal Pharmaceutical Society has been reproduced below and is available online in appendix M of the RPS Governance Handbook (**www.rpharms.com/assembly-pdfs/ governancehandbook.pdf**).

Members will:

- exercise their professional skills and judgement to the best of their ability and discharge their professional responsibilities with integrity considering, where appropriate, the public interest, serving as an example to others;

- do all in their power to ensure that their professional activities do not put the health and safety of others at risk;

- when called upon to give a professional opinion, do so with objectivity and reliability;

- never engage in any corrupt or unethical practice;

- never engage in any activity that will impair the dignity, reputation and welfare of the Society, fellow members or their profession;

- observe the principles of the Statement of Dignity and Respect, set out in appendix U of the Governance Handbook (**http://www.rpharms.com/ assembly-pdfs/governancehandbook.pdf**), when dealing with employees of the Society or their fellow members, members of governing bodies, or members of the public.

7. EXCLUDED TOPICS AND SIGNPOSTING

For some of the topics which have become less relevant to day-to-day pharmacy practice, and are no longer core within the new MEP, the following sources of information may be useful.

TABLE 19: EXCLUDED TOPICS AND SIGNPOSTING

TOPIC	REASON FOR EXCLUSION	ALTERNATIVE RESOURCE
HUMAN A-Z LIST OF MEDICINES	Limited use in day-to-day practice as information is available by marketing authorisation on the packaging of the medicine. Lists are not exhaustive and information exists elsewhere	**RPS website:** remains available to members via online database and PDF **BNF:** CD Schedule information and partial classification for medicines within formulary **MHRA:** Rama XL resource. Commercial access to comprehensive MHRA sentinel database. Available under subscription **Other:** C&D price list, OTC directories, Summary of Product Characteristics database (**www.medicines.org.uk**), Home Office list of Controlled Drugs (**www.gov.uk/government/organisations/home-office**)
LISTS DERIVED FROM MEDICINES LEGISLATION E.G. WHOLESALE LISTS CONDITIONS UNDER WHICH SMALLPOX VACCINE CAN BE ADMINISTERED	Reproduction of legislation and lists from legislation is not a core role of a professional body Some lists are of little relevance to daily practice Alternative sources of information are also available	Human Medicines Regulations 2012 (**www.legislation.gov.uk**) **Appelbe GE, Wingfield J**, editors. *Dale and Applebe's Pharmacy and Medicines Law.* 10th edition. London: Pharmaceutical Press; 2013.
COSHH REGULATIONS	Comprehensive alternative source of information available	Comprehensive information available from the Health and Safety Executive. (**www.hse.gov.uk/coshh**)
DENATURED ALCOHOL	Comprehensive alternative source of information available	Detailed information available in HMRC Notice 473 (**www.gov.uk/government/publications/excise-notice-473-production-distribution-and-use-of-denatured-alcohol**) **Appelbe GE, Wingfield J**, editors. *Dale and Applebe's Pharmacy and Medicines Law.* 10th edition. London: Pharmaceutical Press; 2013.

TOPIC	REASON FOR EXCLUSION	ALTERNATIVE RESOURCE
VETERINARY A-Z LIST OF MEDICINES	Reliable and robust alternative sources of information freely available	Veterinary Medicines Directorate product database (**www.vmd.defra.gov.uk/ ProductInformationDatabase/**) NOAH compendium database (**www.noah.co.uk**)
COMMUNITY PHARMACY CONTRACTUAL FRAMEWORK	Comprehensive alternative source of information available	**England:** Pharmaceutical Services Negotiating Committee (PSNC) (**www.psnc.org.uk**) NHS Community Pharmacy Contractual Framework Service Development (England) (**www.rpharms.com**) **Wales:** Community Pharmacy Wales (**www.cpwales.org.uk**) NHS Community Pharmacy Contractual Framework Service Development (Wales) (**www.rpharms.com**) **Scotland:** Community Pharmacy Scotland (**www.communitypharmacyscotland.org.uk**)
SPECIALS/UNLICENSED MEDICINES	Comprehensive information available on RPS website and alternative source	**RPS:** *Professional Guidance for the Procurement and Supply of Specials.* December 2015. (**www.rpharms.com**) **RPS:** Advice/clarification on crushing tablets and opening capsules. June 2011 (**www.rpharms.com**) **RPS:** Information on pharmaceutical issues when crushing, opening or splitting oral dosage forms (**www.rpharms.com**) **GPhC.** Guidance for registered pharmacies preparing unlicensed medicines **see Appendix 12** or **www.pharmacyregulation.org**
HEALTH AND SAFETY	Comprehensive alternative source of information available	Health and Safety Executive (**www.hse.gov.uk**) **Appelbe GE, Wingfield J**, editors. *Dale and Applebe's Pharmacy and Medicines Law.* 10th edition. London: Pharmaceutical Press; 2013.

8. PARTNERSHIPS WITH SPECIALIST GROUPS

The Royal Pharmaceutical Society is committed to collaborating and co-operating with partners from across the profession to advance pharmacy. We work in partnership with a wide range of specialist groups, many of whom have established networks, to ensure their specialist expertise and knowledge influences and informs the work of the RPS. We work with our partnership groups to ensure a strong voice for the profession and professional support and development for pharmacists working in all areas of pharmacy.

The following table contains details of the partners of the Royal Pharmaceutical Society, some brief information about each group and website details.

TABLE 20: SPECIALIST PARTNERSHIP GROUPS

PARTNERSHIP GROUP	ABOUT OUR PARTNER	DETAILS
AMBULANCE PHARMACISTS NETWORK (APN)	The Ambulance Pharmacists Network meets four times a year and is an opportunity for pharmacists working for ambulance services across the UK to share good medicines management practice	**www.rpharms.com/ sector-groups/ambulance- pharmacists-network.as**p
ASSOCIATION OF PHARMACY TECHNICIANS (APTUK)	The Association of Pharmacy Technicians UK is the professional leadership body for pharmacy technicians working in the UK. The APTUK aims to work on behalf of pharmacy technicians and in partnership with other pharmacy organisations to help deliver professional excellence	**www.aptuk.org**
BRITISH ONCOLOGY PHARMACY ASSOCIATION (BOPA)	BOPA is the British Oncology Pharmacy Association and was formed to 'promote excellence in the pharmaceutical care of patients with cancer through education, communication, research and innovation by an alliance of hospital, community and academic pharmacists, pharmacy technicians, those in the pharmaceutical industry and other healthcare professionals'	**www.bopawebsite.org**
BRITISH PHARMACEUTICAL NUTRITION GROUP (BPNG)	A network for pharmacists, pharmacy technicians, scientists and other healthcare professions with a specialism or interest in any aspect of nutrition, in particular parenteral or enteral nutrition. The aim of the group is to promote and develop best standards within nutrition and to provide high quality education on the subject	**www.bpng.co.uk**

PARTNERSHIP GROUP	ABOUT OUR PARTNER	DETAILS
BRITISH SOCIETY FOR THE HISTORY OF PHARMACY (BSHP)	The British Society for the History of Pharmacy was formed in 1967 having originated from a committee of the Royal Pharmaceutical Society. It seeks to act as a focus for the development of all areas of the history of pharmacy, from the works of the ancient apothecary to today's ever changing role of the community, wholesale or industrial pharmacist	**www.bshp.org**
COLLEGE OF MENTAL HEALTH PHARMACY (CMHP)	The College of Mental Health Pharmacy promotes its members as recognised experts in the optimal use of medicines in improving mental health and supports them by a process of ongoing accreditation and education	**www.cmhp.org.uk**
FACULTY OF CANCER PHARMACY (FCP)	The Faculty is a distinct, autonomous, professional body. It provides professional support for pharmacists in the UK, from any professional background, who are interested and/or working in the specialist area of cancer pharmacy. Launched in January 2008 as a joint venture between the college and The British Oncology Pharmacy Association, it is run by a working board consisting of six people elected from the membership, and works to a formal constitution	**www.rpharms.com/clinical-and-pharmacy-practice/ faculty-of-cancer-pharmacy.asp**
HIV PHARMACISTS ASSOCIATION (HIVPA)	HIVPA is the UK HIV Pharmacy Association which was established in 1991 and has a long history of providing high quality education, support and networking for its members to improve professional and personal development. Its membership is open to all pharmacists and technicians working in or with an interest in HIV, infectious diseases and sexual health. HIVPA organises four highly educational study days with online live streaming and a two-day national conference every year. HIVPA's aim is to promote excellence in the pharmaceutical care of patients living with HIV. HIVPA recognises and promotes advanced pharmacy practice and supports research and collaboration with other healthcare professionals. HIVPA works closely with national HIV charities, campaigns and with the British HIV Association and is represented on several sub committees, e.g. national treatment guidelines and contributes to the national standard documents	**www.hivpa.org**

TABLE 20: SPECIALIST PARTNERSHIP GROUPS (CONTINUED)

PARTNERSHIP GROUP	ABOUT OUR PARTNER	DETAILS
INSTITUTE OF PHARMACY MANAGEMENT (IPM)	The Institute of Pharmacy Management promotes education, research and excellence in pharmacy management. Incorporated in 1964 under the Companies Act as a Limited Company (By Guarantee), the Institute is essentially an educational body which is non-profit making. The Institute embraces all branches of pharmacy: community, hospital, academia, the pharmaceutical industry and wholesale distribution; 10% of its 300 members live in some 20 countries outside the United Kingdom. Membership details can be found on our website	www.ipmi.org.uk
JOINT PHARMACEUTICAL ANALYSIS GROUP (JPAG)	The remit of JPAG is to 'encourage, assist and extend the knowledge and study of pharmaceutical analysis and quality control by the holding of scientific meetings, the promotion of lectures, practical demonstrations and discussions, or by any means consistent with the objectives of the sponsoring bodies and the rules of the Group'. JPAG has close contact with the industrial, academic, NHS and regulatory and enforcement sectors, and serves as the primary UK focus for those with an interest in any aspect of pharmaceutical analysis and related facets of medicines control and registration	www.rpharms.com/science-research-and-technology/ joint-pharmaceutical-analysis-group.asp
NATIONAL ASSOCIATION OF WOMEN PHARMACISTS (NAWP)	The National Association of Women Pharmacists was formed in June 1905 and has the mission of enabling all women pharmacists to realise their full potential and raise their profile by being educationally, socially and politically active. Membership is open to all UK pharmacists and former pharmacists (e.g. retired or taking a career break) and all UK pharmacy graduates, regardless of age or gender. UK undergraduate pharmacy students can join free of charge	www.nawp.org.uk

PARTNERSHIP GROUP	ABOUT OUR PARTNER	DETAILS
NATIONAL PHARMACY CLINICAL TRIALS ADVISORY GROUP (NPCTAG)	The National Pharmacy Clinical Trials Advisory Group (NPCTAG), originally a subgroup of the National Pharmaceutical Quality Assurance Committee, was established in its current form in 2010. Membership of NPCTAG includes representatives from a range of hospital pharmacy disciplines and other relevant specialist groups, MHRA and the National Institute of Health Research. The group's objectives are to: ■ Provide advice to NHS pharmacy services and to the National Institute of Health Research Clinical Research Networks Coordinating Centre ■ Support education and training of pharmacy staff ■ Provide a forum for communication with MHRA about clinical trial issues.	**www.rpharms.com/clinical-and-pharmacy-practice/clinical-trials-network---npctag.asp**
NEONATAL AND PAEDIATRIC PHARMACY GROUP (NPPG)	The Neonatal and Paediatric Pharmacy Group (NPPG) was formed in 1994, with an aim to improve the care of neonates, infants and children by advancing the personal development of pharmacists and technicians through the provision of quality pharmacy services in relation to practice, research and audit, education and training, communication and advice	**www.nppg.org.uk**
PALLIATIVE CARE PHARMACISTS NETWORK (PCPN)	Membership of the Network is open to pharmacists with an interest in palliative care working in hospices, hospitals, community pharmacy, clinical commissioning groups, research and academia	**www.pcpn.org.uk**
PHARMACY LAW AND ETHICS ASSOCIATION (PLEA)	The Pharmacy Law and Ethics Association (PLEA) is an independent group for pharmacists who are involved in law and ethics and lawyers or ethicists who are involved in pharmacy. PLEA was founded in 1997 by Professor Joy Wingfield who is the current chairman	**www.plea.org.uk**

PARTNERSHIPS WITH SPECIALIST GROUPS

PARTNERSHIP GROUP	ABOUT OUR PARTNER	DETAILS
PRIMARY AND COMMUNITY CARE PHARMACY NETWORK (PCCPN)	The overarching aim of the PCCPN is to promote the safe and effective use of medicines in community health and social care settings and to ensure that patients and the public obtain the most effective outcome from the safe use of medicines. Their expertise includes understanding provision of community health services and the standards required to a wide range of settings and services including in-patient services, community nursing, school health, outreach teams, residential and day care, and community clinics. They work on behalf of their members to support them with their day-to-day practice, to promote the highest standards of practice and to help influence national policy and strategies affecting those services for which their members are responsible.	www.pccpnetwork.nhs.uk
PRIMARY CARE PHARMACISTS' ASSOCIATION (PCPA)	The Primary Care Pharmacists' Association (PCPA) was established in 1999 for the benefit of all pharmacists with an active interest in primary care pharmacy. The PCPA is now the largest and longest-standing independent organisation dedicated to supporting pharmacists working within primary care.	www.pcpa.org.uk
RADIOPHARMACY GROUP (UKRPG)	The origins of the UK Radiopharmacy Group date from 1976 and an initiative by a small group of practising radiopharmacists to work together for the advancement of radiopharmacy.	www.bnms.org.uk/ukrg/general/ukrg-homepage.html
SECURE ENVIRONMENT PHARMACISTS GROUP (SEPG)	The SEPG is a special interest group for pharmacists providing professional services to prisons and other secure environments in England and Wales. The group is open to all pharmacists directly providing services to, or with organisational responsibility for, medicines management in these locations.	www.rpharms.com/sector-groups/secure-environment-pharmacists-group.asp

PARTNERSHIP GROUP	ABOUT OUR PARTNER	DETAILS
UNITED KINGDOM CLINICAL PHARMACY ASSOCIATION (UKCPA)	The UK Clinical Pharmacy Association (UKCPA) is a member association for clinical pharmacy practitioners. They encourage, support and promote advanced practice in pharmacy. The UKCPA actively develops clinical pharmacy practice as well as developing individual practitioners, and are frequently at the forefront of initiatives such as establishing professional curricula, developing professional recognition (credentialing) processes, and developing professional tools and frameworks for practitioners.

The Association was established in 1981 with the aim of bringing together like-minded pharmacists from different practice areas to share knowledge, research and experiences. This remains their core aim today. They provide networking and educational opportunities for their members to discuss and resolve current clinical issues and share best practice.

In April 2011 the UKCPA became an official partner of the pharmacy professional body, the Royal Pharmaceutical Society and work closely with other specialist pharmacy organisations, professional bodies and representatives of healthcare professions. | www.ukcpa.net |
| UNITED KINGDOM MEDICINES INFORMATION (UKMi) | UKMi is the United Kingdom Medicines Information network – a pharmacist-led service that helps patients and healthcare professionals working in all sectors to use medicines safely and effectively. They provide evidence-based, tailored advice on the pharmaceutical care of individual patients; they also produce a portfolio of innovative products designed to help clinicians, managers, and commissioners deliver high-quality cost-effective services.

UKMi is a virtual network in which local patient-focused services in acute Trusts are advanced, developed, and supported regionally and nationally. There are around 220 local medicines information centres facilitated by 16 larger ones serving specific geographies; centres pool resource to work under the UKMi banner. National standards underpin the work of medicines information pharmacists and pharmacy technicians, who have both clinical expertise and particular skills in locating and interpreting information about medicines. Through UKMi, pharmacists and pharmacy technicians have access to various training resources and short courses, an active discussion forum, and both regional and national development and networking events. | www.ukmi.nhs.uk |

TABLE 20: SPECIALIST PARTNERSHIP GROUPS (CONTINUED)

PARTNERSHIP GROUP	ABOUT OUR PARTNER	DETAILS
UK OPHTHALMIC PHARMACY GROUP (UKOPG)	The UK Ophthalmic Pharmacy Group aim to promote and develop ophthalmic care within pharmacy, particularly in the hospital setting. The Group develop members' knowledge of the ophthalmology specialty, and discuss and share experiences in ophthalmic care.	www.networks.nhs.uk/ nhs-networks/ophthalmic- pharmacists-group
UNITED KINGDOM RENAL PHARMACY GROUP (UKRPG)	The UK Renal Pharmacy Group (UKRPG) aims to promote excellence in the provision of pharmaceutical services to renal patients and associated healthcare professionals. To this end the Renal Pharmacy Group (UKRPG) publishes and encourages the dissemination of relevant information amongst pharmacists, pharmacy technicians, students and associated healthcare professionals, working in partnership with pharmacy colleagues from other specialties. The UKRPG also actively contributes to, and promotes, pharmaceutical research, audit and innovation in renal medicine and pharmacy practice.	www.renalpharmacy.org. uk/index.php

MEDICINES, ETHICS AND PRACTICE

9. PHARMACIST SUPPORT

Pharmacist Support is an independent charity providing a range of free and confidential support services to pharmacists and their families, former pharmacists, pre-registration trainees and MPharm students in times of need. Services include:

- Information and enquiry service
- Wardley wellbeing service – resources to help manage wellbeing
- Listening Friends – a confidential helpline staffed by trained volunteer pharmacists
- Financial assistance – provided to assist with a range of situations for those experiencing hardship
- Specialist advice in the areas of debt, benefits and employment law
- Addiction support through our Health Support Programme – to assist pharmacists experiencing problems with alcohol, drugs, or other types of dependency.

To discuss your situation and the support available to you in more detail call: 0808 168 2233.

Alternatively you can email the support team on **info@pharmacistsupport.org**

- To speak with a Listening Friend call: 0808 168 5133
- To speak with an addiction specialist call: 0808 168 5132.

All enquiries will be dealt with in confidence.

Further information can be found on the Pharmacist Support website at: **www.pharmacistsupport.org**

APPENDICES

Appendices 1 to 13 are standards and guidance that have been reproduced with the kind permission of the General Pharmaceutical Council (GPhC). These documents are subject to change and review by the GPhC and the latest versions can be obtained from the GPhC website **(www.pharmacyregulation.org)**.

The following additional standards and guidance have not been reproduced in the appendices and can be obtained from the GPhC website **(www.pharmacyregulation.org)**:

■ GPhC Standards for the initial education and training of pharmacists (May 2011)

■ GPhC Standards for the education and training of non-EEA pharmacists wanting to register in Great Britain (May 2011)

■ GPhC Standards for the initial education and training of pharmacy technicians (September 2010)

■ GPhC Guidance on tutoring for pharmacists and pharmacy technicians (January 2014)

■ GPhC Good decision making: fitness to practise hearings and sanctions guidance (July 2015)

■ Joint Statement from the Chief Executives of statutory regulators of healthcare professional. Openness and honesty – the professional duty of candour.

The GPhC Standards Team can be contacted at:

Standards Team
General Pharmaceutical Council
25 Canada Square
London
E14 5LQ

Tel: 020 3713 8000
Email: standards@pharmacyregulation.org

APPENDICES

NB: These appendices have been reproduced with the permission of the GPhC.
Any reference to 'we' or 'us' refers to the GPhC. The material contained within the appendices are copyright
to the GPhC.

APPENDIX 1: GPhC STANDARDS OF CONDUCT, ETHICS AND PERFORMANCE

*At the time of writing GPhC were consulting on new standards for pharmacy professionals that it is anticipated will replace these standards of conduct, ethics and performance. Further information on the new standards can be found on the GPhC website (**www.pharmacyregulation.org**).*

July 2012

This document sets out the standards of conduct, ethics and performance that pharmacy professionals must follow. Pharmacy professionals are pharmacists and pharmacy technicians who are registered with us. It is important that you meet our standards and that you are able to practise safely and effectively. Your conduct will be judged against the standards and failure to comply could put your registration at risk. If someone raises concerns about you we will consider these standards when deciding if we need to take any action. The work of a pharmacy professional can take many forms and you may work in different settings, including clinical practice, education, research and industry.

If you are a pharmacy professional these standards apply to you, even if you do not treat, care for or interact directly with patients and the public. As well as standards of conduct, ethics and performance, we publish other standards which you need to consider together with these standards. To help you to understand these standards, we have published a glossary of terms. We will also publish guidance to advise you on what you will need to do to meet these standards. The glossary and our guidance can be found on our website at: **www.pharmacyregulation.org**

The Seven Principles

As a pharmacy professional, you must:

1. Make patients your first concern.
2. Use your professional judgement in the interests of patients and the public.
3. Show respect for others.
4. Encourage patients and the public to participate in decisions about their care.
5. Develop your professional knowledge and competence.
6. Be honest and trustworthy.
7. Take responsibility for your working practices.

Meeting the standards

We do not dictate how you should meet our standards. Each standard can normally be met in more than one way and the way in which you meet our standards may change over time. The standards are of equal importance. You are professionally accountable for your practice. This means that you are responsible for what you do or do not do, no matter what advice or direction your manager or another professional gives you. You must use your professional judgement when deciding on a course of action and you should use our standards as a basis when making those decisions. You may be faced with conflicting professional or legal responsibilities. In these circumstances you must consider all possible courses of action and the risks and benefits associated with each one to decide what is in the best interests of patients and the public.

1. MAKE PATIENTS YOUR FIRST CONCERN

The care, well-being and safety of patients are at the heart of professional practice. They must always be your first concern. Even if you do not have direct contact with patients your decisions or behaviour can still affect their care or safety.

YOU MUST:

1.1 Make sure the services you provide are safe and of acceptable quality.

1.2 Take action to protect the wellbeing of patients and the public.

1.3 Promote the health of patients and the public.

1.4 Get all the information you require to assess a person's needs in order to give the appropriate treatment and care.

1.5 If you need to, refer patients to other health or social care professionals, or to other relevant organisations.

1.6 Do your best to provide medicines and other professional services safely and when patients need them.

1.7 Be satisfied that patients or their carers know how to use their medicines.

1.8 Keep full and accurate records of the professional services you provide in a clear and legible form.

1.9 Make sure you have access to the facilities, equipment and resources you need to provide your professional services safely and effectively.

1.10 Organise regular reviews, audits and risk assessments to protect patient and public safety and to improve your professional services.

2. USE YOUR PROFESSIONAL JUDGEMENT IN THE INTERESTS OF PATIENTS AND THE PUBLIC

Balancing the needs of individuals with those of society as a whole is essential to professional practice.

YOU MUST:

2.1 Consider and act in the best interests of individual patients and the public.

2.2 Make sure that your professional judgement is not affected by personal or organisational interests, incentives, targets or similar measures.

2.3 Make the best use of the resources available to you.

2.4 Be prepared to challenge the judgement of your colleagues and other professionals if you have reason to believe that their decisions could affect the safety or care of others.

2.5 In an emergency, consider all available options and do your best to provide care and reduce risks to patients and the public.

3. SHOW RESPECT FOR OTHERS

Showing respect for other people is essential in forming and maintaining professional relationships.

YOU MUST:

3.1 Recognise diversity and respect people's cultural differences and their right to hold their personal values and beliefs.

3.2 Treat people politely and considerately.

3.3 Not unfairly discriminate against people. Make sure your views about a person's lifestyle, religion or belief, race, gender reassignment, identity, sex and sexual orientation, age, disability, marital status or any other factors, do not affect how you provide your professional services.

3.4 Make sure that if your religious or moral beliefs prevent you from providing a service, you tell the relevant people or authorities and refer patients and the public to other providers.

3.5 Respect and protect people's dignity and privacy. Take all reasonable steps to prevent accidental disclosure or unauthorised access to confidential information. Never disclose confidential information without consent unless required to do so by the law or in exceptional circumstances.

3.6 Get consent for the professional services you provide and the patient information you use.

3.7 Use information you obtain in the course of your professional practice only for the purposes you were given it, or where the law says you can.

3.8 Make sure you provide the appropriate levels of privacy for patient consultations.

3.9 Maintain proper professional boundaries in your relationships with patients and others that you come into contact with during the course of your professional practice and take special care when dealing with vulnerable people.

4. ENCOURAGE PATIENTS AND THE PUBLIC TO PARTICIPATE IN DECISIONS ABOUT THEIR CARE

Patients and the public have a right to be involved in decisions about their treatment and care. This needs effective communication. You should encourage patients and the public to work in partnership with you and others to manage their needs.

YOU MUST:

4.1 Communicate effectively with patients and the public and take reasonable steps to meet their communication needs.

4.2 Work in partnership with patients and the public, their carers and other professionals to manage their treatment and care. Listen to patients and the public and respect their choices.

4.3 Explain the options available to patients and the public, including the risks and benefits, to help them make informed decisions. Make sure the information you give is impartial, relevant and up to date.

4.4 Respect a person's right to refuse to receive a professional service.

4.5 Make sure that information is appropriately shared with other health and social care professionals involved in the care of the patient.

4.6 Consider and take steps, when possible, to address those factors that may be preventing or deterring patients from getting or taking their treatment.

4.7 If a person cannot legally make decisions about their care, make sure that any service you provide is in line with the appropriate legal requirements.

5. DEVELOP YOUR PROFESSIONAL KNOWLEDGE AND COMPETENCE

Up-to-date and relevant professional knowledge and skills are essential for safe and effective practice. You must ensure that your knowledge, skills and performance are of a high standard, up to date and relevant to your field of practice at all stages of your professional working life.

YOU MUST:

5.1 Recognise the limits of your professional competence. Practise only in those areas in which you are competent to do so and refer to others if you need to.

5.2 Maintain and improve the quality of your practice by keeping your knowledge and skills up to date and relevant to your role and responsibilities.

5.3 Apply your knowledge and skills appropriately to your practice.

5.4 Learn from assessments, appraisals and reviews of your professional performance and undertake further education and training if necessary.

5.5 Undertake and keep up-to-date evidence of your continuing professional development.

6. BE HONEST AND TRUSTWORTHY

Patients and the public put their trust in pharmacy professionals. You must behave in a way that justifies this trust and maintains the reputation of your profession.

YOU MUST:

6.1 Act with honesty and integrity to maintain public trust and confidence in your profession.

6.2 Not abuse your professional position or exploit the vulnerability or lack of knowledge of others.

6.3 Avoid conflicts of interest and declare any personal or professional interests you have. Do not ask for or accept gifts, rewards or hospitality that may affect, or be seen to affect, your professional judgement.

6.4 Be accurate and impartial when you teach and when you provide or publish information. Do not mislead or make claims that you have no evidence for or cannot justify.

6.5 Meet accepted standards of personal and professional conduct.

6.6 Comply with legal and professional requirements and accepted guidance on professional practice.

6.7 Keep to your commitments, agreements and arrangements to provide professional services.

6.8 Respond honestly, openly and politely to complaints and criticism.

6.9 Promptly tell us, your employer and all relevant authorities about anything that may mean you are not fit to practise or that may damage the reputation of the pharmacy professions. This includes ill health that affects your ability to practise, criminal convictions and findings of other regulatory bodies or organisations.

7. TAKE RESPONSIBILITY FOR YOUR WORKING PRACTICES

Working in a team is an important part of professional practice and relies on respect, co-operation and communication between colleagues from your own and other professions. When you work as part of a team you are accountable for your own decisions and behaviour and any work you supervise.

YOU MUST:

7.1 Practise only if you are fit to do so.

7.2 Make sure that you and everyone you are responsible for have the language skills to communicate and work effectively with colleagues.

7.3 Contribute to the development, education and training of colleagues and students, and share your knowledge, skills and expertise.

7.4 Take responsibility for all work you do or are responsible for. Make sure that you delegate tasks only to people who are trained to do them, or who are being trained.

7.5 Make sure it is clear who is responsible for providing a particular service when you are working in a team.

7.6 Be satisfied that appropriate standard operating procedures are in place and are being followed.

7.7 Make sure that you keep to your legal and professional responsibilities and that your workload or working conditions do not present a risk to patient care or public safety.

7.8 Make sure that your actions do not stop others from keeping to their legal and professional responsibilities, or present a risk to patient care or public safety.

7.9 Make sure that all your work, or work that you are responsible for, is covered by appropriate professional indemnity cover.

7.10 Make sure that there is an effective complaints procedure where you work and follow it at all times.

7.11 Make the relevant authority aware of any policies, systems, working conditions, or the actions, professional performance or health of others if they may affect patient care or public safety. If something goes wrong or if someone reports a concern to you, make sure that you deal with it appropriately.

7.12 Co-operate with any investigations into your or another healthcare professional's fitness to practise and keep to undertakings you give or any restrictions placed on your practice because of an investigation.

APPENDIX 2: GPhC STANDARDS FOR REGISTERED PHARMACIES

September 2012

The purpose of these standards is to create and maintain the right environment, both organisational and physical, for the safe and effective practice of pharmacy. The standards apply to all pharmacies registered with the General Pharmaceutical Council.

We recognise that for anyone operating a registered pharmacy there will always be competing demands. These may be professional, managerial, legal or commercial. However, medicines are not ordinary items of commerce. Along with pharmacy services, the supply of medicines is a fundamental healthcare service. Pharmacy owners and superintendent pharmacists must take account of this when applying these standards.

Responsibility for meeting the standards lies with the pharmacy owner. If the registered pharmacy is owned by a 'body corporate' (for example a company or NHS organisation) the superintendent pharmacist also carries responsibility. Pharmacy owners and superintendent pharmacists have the same set of responsibilities; a corporate owner does not avoid responsibility by employing a superintendent. Both are fully responsible for making sure that the standards are met. All those responsible need to take into account the nature of the pharmacy and the services provided and, most importantly, the needs of patients and the public. We also expect them to be familiar with all relevant guidance.

As well as meeting our standards, the pharmacy owner and superintendent pharmacist must make sure they comply with all legal requirements including those covering medicines legislation, health and safety, employment, data protection and equalities legislation.

Pharmacy owners and superintendent pharmacists must make sure that all staff, including non-pharmacists, involved in the management of pharmacy services are familiar with the standards and understand the importance of their being met. All registered professionals working in a registered pharmacy should also be familiar with these standards; and pharmacists and pharmacy technicians must understand that they have a professional responsibility to raise concerns if they believe the standards are not being met.

The standards can also be used by patients and the public so that they know what they should expect when they receive pharmacy services from registered pharmacies.

Throughout this document we use the term 'pharmacy services'. This covers all pharmacy-related services provided by a registered pharmacy including the management of medicines, provision of advice and referral, clinical services such as vaccination services, and services provided to care homes.

Throughout this document we use the term 'staff'. This includes agency and contract workers, as well as employees and other people who are involved in the provision of pharmacy services by a registered pharmacy.

In this document we use the term 'you'. This means:

- A pharmacist who owns a pharmacy as a sole trader, and
- A pharmacist who owns a pharmacy as a partner in a partnership, and
- A pharmacist who is the appointed superintendent pharmacist for a body corporate, and
- The body corporate itself.

In some limited circumstances (for example following death or bankruptcy), a representative can take the role of the pharmacy owner. In these cases, the appointed representative will be responsible for making sure these standards are met.

STANDARDS FOR REGISTERED PHARMACIES

We have grouped the standards under five principles. The principles are the backbone of our regulatory approach and are all equally important.

THE PRINCIPLES

Principle 1: The governance arrangements safeguard the health, safety and wellbeing of patients and the public.

Principle 2: Staff are empowered and competent to safeguard the health, safety and wellbeing of patients and the public.

Principle 3: The environment and condition of the premises from which pharmacy services are provided, and any associated premises, safeguard the health, safety and wellbeing of patients and the public.

Principle 4: The way in which pharmacy services, including the management of medicines and medical devices, are delivered safeguards the health, safety and wellbeing of patients and the public.

Principle 5: The equipment and facilities used in the provision of pharmacy services safeguard the health, safety and wellbeing of patients and the public.

THE STANDARDS

The standards under each principle are requirements that must be met when you operate a registered pharmacy.

Responsibility for meeting the standards lies with the pharmacy owner. If the registered pharmacy is owned by a 'body corporate' (for example, a company or NHS organisation) the superintendent pharmacist also carries responsibility. Pharmacy owners and superintendent pharmacists have the same set of responsibilities; a corporate owner does not avoid responsibility by employing a superintendent. Both are fully responsible for making sure that the standards are met.

If a registered pharmacy is owned by a body corporate, the superintendent must have the authority to:

- Comply with their professional and legal obligations, and
- Use their professional judgement in the best interests of patients and the public.

APPLYING THE STANDARDS

The principles for registered pharmacies, and the standards that must be met, are all equally important. Therefore you should read all the standards in their entirety. Pharmacy owners, superintendent pharmacists and other pharmacy professionals should also be familiar with the standards of conduct, ethics and performance.

We know that a pharmacy owner and superintendent pharmacist may be accountable for one, a few or a large number of registered pharmacies. We expect the pharmacy owner and superintendent pharmacist to make sure that these standards are met whatever the number of pharmacies they are accountable for.

PRINCIPLE 1:

The governance arrangements safeguard the health, safety and wellbeing of patients and the public.

'Governance arrangements' includes having clear definitions of the roles and accountabilities of the people involved in providing and managing pharmacy services.

It also includes the arrangements for managing risks, and the way the registered pharmacy is managed and operated.

STANDARDS

1.1 The risks associated with providing pharmacy services are identified and managed.

1.2 The safety and quality of pharmacy services are reviewed and monitored.

1.3 Pharmacy services are provided by staff with clearly defined roles and clear lines of accountability.

1.4 Feedback and concerns about the pharmacy, services and staff can be raised by individuals and organisations, and these are taken into account and action taken where appropriate.

1.5 Appropriate indemnity or insurance arrangements are in place for the pharmacy services provided.

1.6 All necessary records for the safe provision of pharmacy services are kept and maintained.

1.7 Information is managed to protect the privacy, dignity and confidentiality of patients and the public who receive pharmacy services.

1.8 Children and vulnerable adults are safeguarded.

PRINCIPLE 2:

Staff are empowered and competent to safeguard the health, safety and wellbeing of patients and the public.

The staff you employ and the people you work with are key to the safe and effective practice of pharmacy. Staff members, and anyone involved in providing pharmacy services, must be competent and empowered to safeguard the health, safety and wellbeing of patients and the public in all that they do.

STANDARDS

2.1 There are enough staff, suitably qualified and skilled, for the safe and effective provision of the pharmacy services provided.

2.2 Staff have the appropriate skills, qualifications and competence for their role and the tasks they carry out, or are working under the supervision of another person while they are in training.

2.3 Staff can comply with their own professional and legal obligations and are empowered to exercise their professional judgement in the interests of patients and the public.

2.4 There is a culture of openness, honesty and learning.

2.5 Staff are empowered to provide feedback and raise concerns about meeting these standards and other aspects of pharmacy services.

2.6 Incentives or targets do not compromise the health, safety or wellbeing of patients and the public, or the professional judgement of staff.

PRINCIPLE 3:

The environment and condition of the premises from which pharmacy services are provided, and any associated premises, safeguard the health, safety and wellbeing of patients and the public.

It is important that patients and the public receive pharmacy services from premises that are suitable for the services being provided and which protect and maintain their health, safety and wellbeing. To achieve this you must make sure that all premises where pharmacy services are provided are safe and suitable. Any associated premises, for example non-registered premises used to store medicines, must also comply with these standards where applicable.

STANDARDS

3.1 Premises are safe, clean, properly maintained and suitable for the pharmacy services provided.

3.2 Premises protect the privacy, dignity and confidentiality of patients and the public who receive pharmacy services.

3.3 Premises are maintained to a level of hygiene appropriate to the pharmacy services provided.

3.4 Premises are secure and safeguarded from unauthorised access.

3.5 Pharmacy services are provided in an environment that is appropriate for the provision of healthcare.

PRINCIPLE 4:

The way in which pharmacy services, including the management of medicines and medical devices, are delivered safeguards the health, safety and wellbeing of patients and the public.

'Pharmacy services' covers all pharmacy-related services provided by a registered pharmacy including the management of medicines, advice and referral, and the wide range of clinical services pharmacies provide. The management of medicines includes arrangements for obtaining, keeping, handling, using and supplying medicinal products and medical devices, as well as security and waste management.

Medicines and medical devices are not ordinary commercial items. The way they are managed is fundamental to ensuring the health, safety and wellbeing of patients and the public who receive pharmacy services.

STANDARDS

4.1 The pharmacy services provided are accessible to patients and the public.

4.2 Pharmacy services are managed and delivered safely and effectively.

4.3 Medicines and medical devices are:

- Obtained from a reputable source
- Safe and fit for purpose
- Stored securely
- Safeguarded from unauthorised access
- Supplied to the patient safely
- Disposed of safely and securely.

4.4 Concerns are raised when it is suspected that medicines or medical devices are not fit for purpose.

PRINCIPLE 5:

The equipment and facilities used in the provision of pharmacy services safeguard the health, safety and wellbeing of patients and the public.

The availability of safe and suitable equipment and facilities is fundamental to the provision of pharmacy services and is essential if staff are to safeguard the health, safety and wellbeing of patients and the public when providing effective pharmacy services.

STANDARDS

5.1 Equipment and facilities needed to provide pharmacy services are readily available.

5.2 Equipment and facilities are:

- Obtained from a reputable source
- Safe to use and fit for purpose
- Stored securely
- Safeguarded from unauthorised access
- Appropriately maintained.

5.3 Equipment and facilities are used in a way that protects the privacy and dignity of the patients and the public who receive pharmacy services.

APPENDIX 3: GPhC STANDARDS FOR CONTINUING PROFESSIONAL DEVELOPMENT

September 2010

This document sets out the standards for continuing professional development (CPD). It is important that you meet our standards and that you are able to practise safely and effectively. The CPD requirements apply equally to all pharmacy professionals. They are not changed by factors such as part-time employment, or working in a position of authority. You are expected to cover the full scope of your practice in your CPD record, including responsibilities such as superintendent or pharmacist prescriber and roles in different settings such as industry and community pharmacy. Your conduct will be judged against the standards and failure to comply could put your registration at risk. If someone raises concerns about you we will consider these standards when deciding if we need to take any action. To help you to understand these standards, we have published a glossary of terms. We will also publish guidance to advise you on what you will need to do to meet these standards. The glossary and our guidance can be found on our website at **www.pharmacyregulation.org**

Patients, the public and government expect that every pharmacy professional maintains their professional capability throughout their career. Keeping a record of your CPD enables you to confirm that you are meeting these expectations. It also helps you to retain and build your confidence as a professional and it will provide evidence that you meet our CPD requirement.

1.1 Keep a record of your CPD that is legible, either electronically online at the website **www.uptodate.org.uk**, on another computer, or as hard copy on paper and in a format published or approved by us and carrying the CPD approved logo.

1.2 Make a minimum of nine CPD entries per year which reflect the context and scope of your practice as a pharmacist or pharmacy technician.

1.3 Keep a record of your CPD that complies with the good practice criteria for CPD recording published in Plan and Record by us (**www.pharmacyregulation.org**).

1.4 Record how your CPD has contributed to the quality or development of your practice using our CPD framework.

1.5 Submit your CPD record to us on request.

APPENDIX 4: GPhC GUIDANCE ON PATIENT CONFIDENTIALITY

April 2012

ABOUT THIS GUIDANCE

This guidance should be read alongside the **standards of conduct, ethics and performance** which all pharmacists and pharmacy technicians must apply to their practice. This document gives guidance on standards 3.5, 3.7 and 3.8 of the standards of conduct, ethics and performance, which say:

■ You must respect and protect people's dignity and privacy. Take all reasonable steps to prevent accidental disclosure or unauthorised access to confidential information. Never disclose confidential information without consent unless required to do so by the law or in exceptional circumstances

■ You must use information you obtain in the course of your professional practice only for the purposes you were given it, or where the law says you can

■ You must make sure you provide the appropriate levels of privacy for patient consultations.

STATUS OF THIS GUIDANCE

This document gives guidance to pharmacy professionals on how to meet the standards on confidentiality. The guidance is not intended to cover every issue and it does not give detailed legal advice. However, it reflects the current law in Great Britain.

You should use your professional judgement in applying this guidance in your own practice. You must make sure that you keep up to date and comply with the law, for example: the Data Protection Act 1998, the Human Rights Act 1998, and the common law duty of confidentiality, and with any NHS or employment policies on confidentiality that apply to your particular area of work.

You must make sure that all staff members you are responsible for are aware of this guidance and appropriately trained in all areas that are relevant to their duties. If you are not sure about what you should do in a specific situation, you should always ask for advice from your employer, your professional indemnity insurance provider, your professional body or other pharmacy organisation, or get independent legal advice.

We have produced more guidance to help pharmacy professionals apply our standards of conduct, ethics and performance. You can find this on our website. In particular, when reading this guidance you should also see our 'Guidance on consent'.

1. DUTY OF CONFIDENTIALITY

1.1 You have a professional and legal duty to keep confidential the information you obtain during the course of your professional practice. Maintaining confidentiality is a vital part of the relationship between a pharmacy professional and a patient. Patients may be reluctant to ask for advice, or give you the information you need to provide proper care, if they believe that you may not keep the information confidential. Your duty of confidentiality applies to everyone whatever their age (see our guidance on consent).

1.2 The duty of confidentiality applies to all information you obtain during the course of your professional practice.

1.3 Confidential information includes:

■ Electronic and hard copy data

■ Personal details

■ Information about a person's medication (prescribed and non-prescribed)

■ Other information about a person's medical history, treatment or care that could identify them, and

■ Information that patients or the public share with you that is not strictly medical in nature.

1.4 Confidential information does not include:

■ Anonymous information – information from which individuals cannot reasonably be identified

■ Coded information – information from which individuals cannot reasonably be identified, but which enables information about different patients to be distinguished (for example to identify drug side effects)

■ Information that is already legitimately in the public domain.

2. PROTECTING INFORMATION

2.1 It is essential that you take steps to protect the confidential information you are given in the course of your professional practice. You must:

- Take all reasonable steps to protect the confidentiality of information you receive, store, send or destroy

- Store hard copy and electronic documents, records, registers, prescriptions and other sources of confidential information securely. Do not leave confidential information where it may be seen or accessed by patients, the public or anyone else who should not have access to it

- Take steps to prevent accidental disclosure of confidential information

- Not discuss information that can identify patients where the discussions can be overheard by others not involved in their care

- Not disclose information on any websites, internet chat forums or social media that could identify a patient

- Make sure that everyone who works in your pharmacy knows about their responsibility to maintain confidentiality

- Raise concerns with the person with responsibility for data control where you work, or with any other appropriate authority, if you find that the security of personal information on the premises where you work is not appropriate

- Continue to protect a person's confidentiality after they have died, subject to disclosures required by law or when it is in the public interest (see below).

3. DISCLOSING CONFIDENTIAL INFORMATION

3.1 Decisions about disclosing confidential information can be complex. In most situations you do not have to disclose information immediately. However, there will be limited situations where to delay is not practical, for example if this may cause risk to another person. You should take the necessary steps to satisfy yourself that any disclosure sought is appropriate and meets the legal requirements covering confidentiality.

3.2 Maintaining confidentiality is an important duty, but there are circumstances when it may be appropriate to disclose confidential patient information. These are:

- When you have the patient's consent, or

- When the law says you must, or

- When it is in the public interest to do so.

3.3 In the course of your professional practice you may receive requests for confidential patient information from a variety of people (for example a patient's relative, partner or carer) or organisations (for example the police or a healthcare regulator). You should make decisions about disclosing information on a case-by-case basis and fully consider all relevant factors.

3.4 If a patient with capacity refuses to give consent for information to be shared with other healthcare professionals involved in providing care, it may mean that the care they can be provided is limited. You must respect their decision, but inform the patient of the potential implications on their care or treatment.

3.5 You must respect the wishes of a patient with capacity who does not consent to information about him or her being shared with others, unless the law says you must disclose the information or it is in the public interest to make such a disclosure.

3.6 If you decide to disclose confidential patient information you should:

- Code the information, or make it anonymous, if you do not need to identify the patient

- Get the patient's consent to share their information. But you do not need to do this if:

  - Disclosure is required by law

  - The disclosure can be justified in the public interest

  - To do so is impracticable, would put you or others at risk of serious harm, or would prejudice the purpose of the disclosure

- Disclose only the information needed for the particular purpose

- Make sure that, if you disclose confidential information, the people receiving the information know that it is confidential and is to be treated as such

- Make appropriate records to show:
  - Who the request came from
  - Whether you obtained the patient's consent, or your reasons for not doing so
  - Whether consent was given or refused, and
  - What you disclosed
- Be prepared to justify your decisions and any actions you take
- Release the information promptly once you are satisfied what information should be disclosed and have taken all necessary steps to protect confidentiality.

3A. DISCLOSING INFORMATION WITH CONSENT

3.7 You should get the patient's consent to share their information unless that would undermine the purpose of disclosure (see Section 3b).

3.8 Make sure the patient understands:
- What information will be disclosed
- Why information will be disclosed
- Who it will be disclosed to
- The likely consequences of disclosing and of not disclosing the information.

3.9 When the reason for sharing confidential patient information is for a purpose that the patient would not reasonably expect, you must get their explicit consent before disclosure.

3.10 If you are not sure whether you have the patient's consent to share their information, you should contact them and obtain their consent.

3B. DISCLOSING INFORMATION WITHOUT CONSENT

3.11 You should make every effort to get consent to disclose confidential information. However, if that would undermine the purpose of disclosure (for example when there is risk to others) or is not practicable, you should use the guidance in this section.

3.12 Before you disclose information without the consent of the patient, you should:

- Be satisfied that the law requires you to disclose the information or that disclosure can be justified as being in the public interest
- Ask for clarification from the person making the request if you are unsure about the basis for the request for confidential information
- Ask for the request in writing.

3.13 If necessary get advice from a relevant body, for example your indemnity insurance provider, union, professional body or other pharmacy organisation, or an independent legal advisor.

DISCLOSURES REQUIRED BY LAW

3.14 There are circumstances when the law may require you to disclose information that you hold. These circumstances include when a person or body is using their powers under the law to ask for the information, for example:

- The police or another enforcement, prosecuting or regulatory authority
- A healthcare regulator, such as ourselves or the GMC
- An NHS counter-fraud investigation officer
- A coroner or procurator fiscal, judge, or relevant court which orders that the information should be disclosed.

3.15 These individuals and organisations do not have an automatic right to access all confidential patient information. You must be satisfied they have a legitimate reason for requesting the information.

3.16 If necessary get advice from a relevant body, for example your indemnity insurance provider, union, professional body or other pharmacy organisation or an independent legal advisor.

DISCLOSURES MADE IN THE PUBLIC INTEREST

3.17 These decisions are complex and must take account of both the patient and public interest in maintaining or breaching confidentiality.

3.18 You may disclose confidential information when you consider it to be in the public interest to do so, for example if the information is required to prevent:

- A serious crime
- Serious harm to a patient or third party, or
- Serious risk to public health.

3.19 You must carefully balance the competing interests of maintaining the confidentiality of the information and the public interest benefit in disclosing the information.

3.20 You must consider the possible harm that may be caused by not disclosing the information against the potential consequences of disclosing the information. This includes considering how disclosing the information may affect the care of the patient and the trust that they have in pharmacy professionals.

3.21 If necessary get advice from a relevant body, for example your indemnity insurance provider, union, professional body or other pharmacy organisation, or independent legal advisor.

4. OTHER SOURCES OF INFORMATION

THE INFORMATION COMMISSIONER'S OFFICE

Tel: 0303 123 1113 or 0162 554 5745

HEAD OFFICE

Wycliffe House
Water Lane
Wilmslow
Cheshire SK9 5AF

SCOTLAND OFFICE

45 Melville Street
Edinburgh EH3 7HL

WALES OFFICE

2nd Floor Churchill House
Churchill Way
Cardiff CF10 2HH

Email: casework@ico.gsi.gov.uk

Website: https://ico.org.uk/

APPENDIX 5: GPhC GUIDANCE ON CONSENT

February 2012

This guidance should be read alongside the **standards of conduct, ethics and performance** which all pharmacists and pharmacy technicians must apply to their practice. This document gives guidance on standard 3.6 of the standards of conduct, ethics and performance, which says:

You must get consent for the professional services you provide and the patient information you use.

This document gives guidance to pharmacy professionals on how to meet the standard of consent. The guidance is not intended to cover every situation and it does not give detailed legal advice. However, it reflects the current law in Great Britain.

Pharmacy professionals work in many different settings, so how relevant this guidance is to you may vary depending on your role and the type of patient contact that you have. You should use your professional judgement in applying this guidance in your own practice. You must make sure that you keep up to date and comply with the law, and with any NHS or employment policies for consent that apply to your particular area of work.

You must make sure that all staff members you are responsible for are aware of this guidance and are appropriately trained in all areas that are relevant to their duties.

If you are not sure about how the law applies in a specific situation, you should always ask for advice from appropriate professional colleagues, your employer, your professional indemnity insurance provider, your professional body or other pharmacy organisation, or get independent legal advice.

We have produced more guidance to help pharmacy professionals apply our standards of conduct, ethics and performance. You can find this on our website. In particular, when reading this guidance you should also see our 'Guidance on patient confidentiality'.

1. CONSENT

1.1 WHAT IS CONSENT?

1.1.1 The Oxford English Dictionary defines 'consent' as 'to express willingness, give permission, agree'.

1.1.2 Patients have a basic right to be involved in decisions about their healthcare. The process of obtaining consent is a fundamental part of respect for patients' rights.

1.1.3 Obtaining consent is also essential in forming and maintaining effective partnerships between you and your patients.

1.1.4 You have a professional and legal duty to get a patient's consent for the professional services, treatment or care you provide, or to use patient information.

1.1.5 You must know and comply with the law and the good practice requirements about consent which apply to you in your day-to-day practice.

1.2 TYPES OF CONSENT

1.2.1 There are two types of consent:

- Explicit (or 'express') consent: when a patient gives you specific permission to do something, either spoken or written

- Implied consent: when a patient indicates their consent indirectly, for example by bringing their prescription to you to be dispensed. This is not a lesser form of consent but it is only valid if the patient knows and understands what they are consenting to. If you are not sure whether you have implied consent, you should get explicit consent.

1.2.2 You must use your professional judgement to decide what type of consent to get. You should take into account legal requirements, NHS service requirements, and policies where you work that may set this out.

1.2.3 When appropriate, you should record the fact that the patient has given explicit consent and what they have consented to.

1.3 OBTAINING CONSENT

1.3.1 For consent to be valid the patient must:

- Have the capacity to give consent
- Be acting voluntarily – they must not be under any undue pressure from you or anyone else to make a decision
- Have sufficient, balanced information to allow them to make an informed decision
- Be capable of using and weighing up the information provided.

1.3.2 The information you provide to the patient must be clear, accurate and presented in a way that the patient can understand. For example, you must consider any disabilities, or literacy or language barriers.

1.3.3 You should not make assumptions about the patient's level of knowledge and you should give them the opportunity to ask questions.

1.3.4 You are responsible for making sure that a patient has given valid consent. You must use your professional judgement to decide whether you should get consent from the patient yourself, or whether this task can be properly delegated. If you do delegate the task you must make sure that you delegate it to a competent and appropriately trained member of staff.

1.3.5 Getting consent is an ongoing process between you and the patient. Consent cannot be presumed just because it was given on a previous occasion. You must get a patient's consent on each occasion that it is needed, for example when there is a change in treatment or service options.

1.3.6 Patients with capacity are entitled to withdraw their consent at any time.

2. CAPACITY

2.1 WHAT IS CAPACITY?

2.1.1 In England and Wales, under the Mental Capacity Act (2005), a person lacks capacity if at the time the decision needs to be made, they are unable to make or communicate the decision, because of an 'impairment or disturbance' that affects the way their mind or brain works.

2.1.2 In Scotland, under the Adults with Incapacity (Scotland) Act (2000), a person lacks capacity if they cannot make decisions or communicate them, or understand or remember their decisions, because of a mental disorder or physical inability to communicate in any form.

2.2 ASSESSING CAPACITY

2.2.1 You must base an assessment of capacity on the patient's ability to make a specific decision at the time it needs to be made. A patient may be capable of making some decisions but not others.

2.2.2 In general, to make an informed decision the patient should be able to:

- Understand the information provided
- Remember the information provided
- Use and weigh up the information provided, and
- Communicate their decision to you (by any means).

2.2.3 You must not assume that because a patient lacks capacity on one occasion, or in relation to one type of service, that they lack capacity to make all decisions.

2.2.4 A patient's capacity to consent may be temporarily affected by other factors, for example fatigue, panic, or the effects of drugs or alcohol. The existence of these factors should not lead to an automatic assumption that the patient does not have the capacity to consent. Instead you should use your professional judgement to make a decision based on the individual circumstances.

2.2.5 You must not assume that a patient lacks capacity based just upon their age, disability, beliefs, condition, or behaviour, or because they make a decision you disagree with.

2.2.6 You must take all reasonable steps to help and support patients to make their own decisions or to be as involved as they can be in a decision. For example:

- Time the discussion for when the patient's understanding may be better
- Use appropriate types of communication, simple language or visual aids
- Get someone else to help with communication such as a family member, support worker or interpreter.

2.2.7 If you are unsure about a patient's capacity you must get advice from other healthcare professionals or people involved in their care.

2.2.8 If you are still unsure you must get legal advice.

2.2.9 Any advice you get or assessments carried out should be properly recorded, along with the outcome.

2.2.10 You can find more guidance on how people should be helped to make their own decisions, and how to assess capacity, in the Codes of Practice that accompany the Mental Capacity Act (2005) and Adults with Incapacity (Scotland) Act (2000).

2.3 ADULTS WITH CAPACITY

2.3.1 Every adult is presumed to have the capacity to make their own decisions (that is, they are competent) and to give consent for a service or treatment unless there is enough evidence to suggest otherwise.

2.4 WHEN A COMPETENT ADULT REFUSES TO GIVE CONSENT

2.4.1 If an adult with capacity makes a voluntary, informed decision to refuse a service or treatment you must respect their decision, even when you think that their decision is wrong or may cause them harm. This does not apply when the law says otherwise, such as when compulsory treatment is authorised by mental health legislation[1].

2.4.2 You should clearly explain the consequences of their decision but you must make sure that you do not pressure the patient to accept your advice.

2.4.3 You should make a detailed record if a patient refuses to give consent. This should include the discussions that have taken place and the advice you gave.

2.4.4 If you believe that the patient is at risk of serious harm due to their decision to refuse a service or treatment, you must raise this issue with appropriate healthcare or pharmacy colleagues or people involved in their care, and your employer (if applicable). Consider getting legal advice if necessary.

[1]Mental Health Act 2003 (as amended by the Mental Health Act 2006), and the Mental Health (Care and Treatment) (Scotland) Act 2003.

2.5 ADULTS WITHOUT CAPACITY

2.5.1 If the patient is not able to make decisions for themselves, you must work with people close to them and with other members of the healthcare team.

2.5.2 The Mental Capacity Act (2005) and Adults with Incapacity (Scotland) Act (2000) set out the criteria and the processes to be followed in making decisions and providing care services when a patient lacks the capacity to make some or all decisions for themselves. They also grant legal authority to certain people to make decisions on behalf of patients who lack capacity.

2.5.3 If you believe that a patient lacks capacity to make decisions for themselves, consult the Codes of Practice that accompany the Mental Capacity Act (2005) or Adults with Incapacity (Scotland) Act (2000). These set out who can make decisions on the patient's behalf, in which situations, and how they should go about this.

2.6 YOUNG PEOPLE AND CHILDREN

2.6.1 The capacity to consent depends more on the patient's ability to understand and consider their decision than on their age.

2.6.2 In this guidance a young person means anyone aged 16 or 17 and a child means anyone aged under 16. However, people gain full legal capacity in relation to medical treatment at a different age in Scotland than in England and Wales.

2.6.3 As with any patient, a young person or child may have the capacity to consent to some services or treatments but not to others. Therefore it is important that you assess maturity and understanding individually, and bearing in mind the complexity and importance of the decision to be made.

2.6.4 If a person with parental responsibility is required to provide consent, you may need to get legal advice if:

- You are in any doubt about who has parental responsibility for the individual, or
- The views of those that have parental responsibility differ.

2.6.5 Young people and children should be involved as much as possible in decisions about their care, even when they are not able to make decisions on their own.

2.7 YOUNG PEOPLE WITH CAPACITY

2.7.1 Young people are presumed to have the capacity to make their own decisions and give consent for a service or treatment, unless there is enough evidence to suggest otherwise.

2.7.2 To decide whether a young person has the capacity to consent to a service or treatment, use the same criteria as for adults (see section 2.2 'Assessing capacity').

2.7.3 You should encourage young people to involve their parents in making important decisions. However, you should respect a competent young person's request for confidentiality.

2.8 CHILDREN WITH CAPACITY

2.8.1 Children are not presumed to have the capacity to consent. They must demonstrate their competence.

2.8.2 A child can give consent if you are satisfied that the treatment is in their best interests, and that they have the maturity and ability to fully understand the information given and what they are consenting to. In this case you do not also need consent from a person with parental responsibility.

2.9 WHEN COMPETENT YOUNG PEOPLE AND CHILDREN REFUSE TO GIVE CONSENT

England and Wales

2.9.1 In some circumstances, the courts can override the refusal of consent of a young person or child. You should get legal advice if needed on this issue.

2.9.2 The law is complex when a competent young person or child refuses to give consent for a treatment or service and someone with parental responsibility wants to override their decision. You should get legal advice if you are faced with this situation.

Scotland

2.9.3 When a young person or child has capacity to make a decision, then the law[2] says that their decision should be respected. This applies even if the decision differs from your view, or from the views of those with parental responsibility.

2.9.4 However, this position has not yet been fully tested in the Scottish courts, and nor has the issue of whether a court can override a young person's or child's decision. You should therefore get legal advice if you are faced with this situation.

[2]*The Age of Legal Capacity (Scotland) Act 1991.*

2.10 YOUNG PEOPLE WITHOUT CAPACITY

England and Wales

2.10.1 A person with parental responsibility for a young person can give consent on behalf of that young person to investigations and treatment that are in the young person's best interests.

Scotland

2.10.2 The rights of a person with parental responsibility to make decisions on behalf of a child ends when the child reaches the age of 16.

2.10.3 Young people who do not have the capacity to consent should be treated as though they are adults and in line with the Adults with Incapacity (Scotland) Act (2000).

2.11 CHILDREN WITHOUT CAPACITY

2.11.1 When a child lacks capacity to give consent, any person with parental responsibility for that child, or the court, can give consent on their behalf.

3. ADVANCE DECISIONS

3.1 People who understand the implications of their choices can say in advance how they want to be treated if they later suffer loss of mental capacity.

3.2 An unambiguous advance refusal for a treatment, procedure or intervention which is voluntarily made by a competent, informed adult is likely to have legal force.

3.3 An advance refusal of treatment cannot override the legal authority to give compulsory treatment under the mental health laws.

3.4 Any advance decision is superseded by a competent decision by the person concerned, given at the time consent is sought.

England and Wales

3.5 Advance decisions are covered by the Mental Capacity Act (2005). For an advance refusal of treatment to be legally valid, it must meet certain criteria set out in the Mental Capacity Act (2005).

3.6 If an advance decision does not meet these criteria, it is not legally binding but can still be used in deciding the patient's best interests.

3.7 You must follow an advance decision if it is valid and applicable to current circumstances.

Scotland

3.8 The Adults with Incapacity (Scotland) Act (2000) does not specifically cover advance decisions. However, it says that health professionals must take account of the patient's past and present wishes, however they were communicated.

3.9 It is likely that you would be bound by a valid and applicable advance decision. However, there have been no specific cases yet considered by the Scottish courts. If in any doubt, get legal advice.

4. EMERGENCIES

4.1 In an emergency, if you cannot get consent, you can provide treatment that is in the patient's best interests and is needed to save their life or prevent deterioration in the patient's condition (this applies to children, young people and adults).

4.2 There is an exception to 4.1 above if you know there is a valid and applicable advance decision to refuse a particular treatment. For more information see the relevant incapacity legislation and its Code of Practice, or ask your professional indemnity insurance provider or a legal advisor.

5. OTHER SOURCES OF INFORMATION

ENGLAND AND WALES

Mental Capacity Act 2005

www.legislation.gov.uk/ukpga/2005/9/contents

Mental Capacity Act Code of Practice

https://www.gov.uk/government/publications/mental-capacity-act-code-of-practice

SCOTLAND

Adults with Incapacity (Scotland) Act 2000

www.legislation.gov.uk/asp/2000/4/contents

Scottish Government site for the Act

www.scotland.gov.uk/Topics/Justice/Civil/awi

APPENDIX 6: GPhC GUIDANCE ON RAISING CONCERNS

February 2012

The issue of raising concerns has been the subject of several high-profile cases in the past twenty years, including the inquiry into Bristol Royal Infirmary and the Shipman Inquiry. The Health Select Committee highlighted in two public reports[i] the importance of healthcare professionals raising concerns. It is therefore important to give pharmacists and pharmacy technicians guidance on this subject. We must make sure that we all learn from past incidents and the experiences of other regulators.

This guidance should be read alongside the **standards of conduct, ethics and performance** which all pharmacists and pharmacy technicians must apply to their practice.

This document gives guidance on standards 1.2, 2.4 and 7.11 of the standards of conduct, ethics and performance, which say:

- You must take action to protect the wellbeing of patients and the public
- You must be prepared to challenge the judgement of your colleagues and other professionals if you have reason to believe that their decisions could affect the safety or care of others
- You must make the relevant authority aware of any policies, systems, working conditions, or the actions, professional performance, or health of others if they may affect patient care or public safety. If something goes wrong or if someone reports a concern to you, make sure that you deal with it appropriately.

This document gives guidance to pharmacy professionals on how to raise concerns. The guidance explains the importance of raising concerns and the steps that a pharmacy professional will need to consider taking.

It also contains extra guidance specifically for employers. You can find the contact details of organisations that may be able to give further support and guidance in section 6 of this document.

You must make sure that you keep up to date with and follow any NHS or employment policies for raising concerns where you practise. You must also make sure that all staff members you are responsible for are aware of this guidance and appropriately trained.

1. THE IMPORTANCE OF RAISING CONCERNS

Every pharmacy professional has a duty to raise any concerns about individuals, actions or circumstances that may be unacceptable and that could result in risks to patient and public safety.

1.1 You have a professional responsibility to take action to protect the wellbeing of patients and the public. Raising concerns about individual pharmacy professionals, the staff you work with (including trainees), employers and the environment you work in is a key part of this.

1.2 This includes raising and reporting any concerns you have about the people you come into contact with during the course of your work, including pharmacists, pharmacy technicians, pharmacy owners, managers and employers, other healthcare professionals or people responsible for the care of a patient, such as carers, care home staff or key workers. It includes concerns about behaviours, competency, the working environment and any actions that may compromise patient safety.

1.3 We recognise that you may be reluctant to raise a concern for a variety of reasons. For example, you may be worried that:

- You will cause trouble for your colleagues
- There may be a negative impact on your career
- It may lead to difficult working relationships with your colleagues
- You could face reprisals
- Nothing will be done as a result of the concern being raised.

Raising concerns at an early stage can help to identify areas of practice that can be improved. It allows employers, regulators and other authorities to take corrective action as quickly as possible and before any direct harm comes to patients and the public.

1.4 You must remember that:

- Your professional duties to safeguard patient and public safety must come before any other loyalties or considerations

- Failing to raise concerns about poor practice could result in harm to patients

- The Public Interest Disclosure Act 1998 (PIDA) protects employees who raise genuine concerns and expose 'malpractice' in the workplace

- If you do not report any concerns you may have about a colleague or others it would be a breach of our standards of conduct, ethics and performance, and this may call into question your own fitness to practise.

2. HOW TO RAISE A CONCERN

How you raise a concern will vary, depending on:

- The nature of your concern

- Who or what you are concerned about, and

- Whether you consider there is a direct or immediate risk of harm to patients or the public.

If you are not sure whether or how to raise your concern you should get advice from one of the organisations listed in section 6.

You have a professional responsibility to raise genuine concerns. You have this responsibility whether you are an employer, employee, a locum or temporary staff.

You should normally raise your concern with your employer first, before taking it to a regulator or other organisation.

2.1 FIND OUT YOUR ORGANISATION'S POLICY

You should find out your employer's policy on raising concerns or 'whistle blowing' and follow this whenever possible.

2.2 REPORT WITHOUT DELAY

If you believe that patients are or may be at risk of death or serious harm you must report your concern without delay.

2.3 REPORT TO YOUR IMMEDIATE SUPERVISOR

The person you report your concerns to will vary depending on the nature of your concern. In most situations, you will be able to raise your concerns with your line manager.

2.4 REPORT TO ANOTHER SUITABLE PERSON IN AUTHORITY OR AN OUTSIDE BODY

There may be some situations when it isn't possible to raise your concerns with your line manager. For example, they may be the cause of your concern or may have strong loyalties to those who are the cause of your concern. In these situations, you may need to speak to:

- A person who has been named as responsible for handling concerns

- A senior manager in the organisation, for example a chief pharmacist, pharmacy owner or superintendent pharmacist or non-pharmacist manager

- The primary care organisation (including the accountable officer if the concern is about Controlled Drugs)

- The health or social care profession regulator[2]

- The relevant systems regulator for the organisation[3].

2.5 KEEP A RECORD

You should keep a record of the concerns you have, who you have raised them with and the response or action that has been taken as a result of your actions.

2.6 MAINTAIN CONFIDENTIALITY

If your concern is about a specific person, for example a patient or colleague, you should, where possible, maintain confidentiality and not disclose information without consent.

3. THE LAW

The PIDA sets out a step-by-step approach to raising and escalating your concern. It aims to protect you from unfair treatment or victimization from your employer if you have made certain disclosures of information in the public interest.

Under the PIDA you should raise a concern about issues which have happened, or which you reasonably believe are likely to happen, and involve:

- A danger to the health or safety of an individual (for example, irresponsible or illegal prescribing, patient abuse, or a professional whose health or fitness to practise may be impaired)

- A crime, or a civil offence (for example, fraud, theft, or the illegal diversion of drugs)
- A miscarriage of justice
- Damage to the environment
- A cover-up of information about any of the above.

This is not a full list. Section 6 gives contact details for other sources of information if you have a concern and you are unsure about whether or how you should raise it.

4. EXTRA GUIDANCE FOR EMPLOYERS

It is important that employees know about the procedures to follow if they have a concern about a colleague or the organisation they work in.

There should also be procedures to identify concerns that should be referred to a regulatory body such as ourselves. Creating an open working environment where your employees feel comfortable raising concerns will safeguard patient safety by helping to identify and therefore improve poor practice.

4.1 Make sure you have fair and robust policies and procedures to manage concerns that are raised with you. These policies and procedures need to be accessible to all staff.

4.2 Encourage all staff, including temporary staff and locums, to raise concerns about the safety of patients, including risks posed by colleagues.

4.3 Make sure that all concerns raised with you are taken seriously and the person who has raised them is not victimised.

4.4 Make sure that all concerns are properly investigated and that all staff, including temporary staff and locums, are kept informed of the progress.

4.5 Have systems in place to give adequate support to pharmacy professionals who have raised concerns, and treat any information you are given in confidence.

4.6 Take appropriate steps to deal with concerns that have been raised because of a failure to maintain standards.

4.7 Have systems in place to support pharmacy professionals who are the subject of the concern, whether it is due to their poor performance, health or behaviour.

4.8 Keep appropriate records of any concerns raised and the actions taken to deal with them.

4.9 Pass records of concerns raised to the manager or superintendent pharmacist so that they can consider an overall assessment of the concerns.

4.10 Do not stop anyone from raising a concern.

5. WHERE TO GO FOR MORE ADVICE

For more information on the PIDA and how to raise your concern under this employment legislation you may want to contact the charity Public Concern at Work (PCaW). This is an independent charity that gives free, confidential legal advice to people who are not sure whether or how to raise concerns about 'malpractice' at work.

If you are not sure whether or how to raise your concern you should get advice from:

- Senior members of staff in your organisation
- The accountable officer, if the concern is about Controlled Drugs
- Your professional indemnity insurance provider, professional body or other pharmacy organisation
- The General Pharmaceutical Council or, if your concern is about a colleague in another healthcare profession, the appropriate regulatory body
- The charity Pharmacist Support
- Your union
- An independent legal advisor.

6. OTHER SOURCES OF INFORMATION

ASSOCIATION OF PHARMACY TECHNICIANS UK

One Victoria Square
Birmingham, B1 1BD
Tel: 020 7121 5551
www.aptuk.org

GUILD OF HEALTHCARE PHARMACISTS

Health Sector, Unite the Union
Unite House, 126 Theobald's Road
London, WC1X 8TN
Tel: 020 3371 2009
www.ghp.org.uk
www.ghpscot.org.uk

NATIONAL PHARMACY ASSOCIATION

Mallinson House, 38-42 St Peter's Street
St Albans AL1 3NP

Tel: 017 2785 8687

www.npa.co.uk

NATIONAL WHISTLEBLOWING HELPLINE

Phone: 0800 0724 725

PHARMACISTS' DEFENCE ASSOCIATION

The Old Fire Station, 69 Albion Street
Birmingham B1 3EA

Tel: 0121 694 7000

www.the-pda.org

PHARMACIST SUPPORT

Tel: 0808 168 2233 (freephone)

www.pharmacistsupport.org

PUBLIC CONCERN AT WORK

Suite 301, 16 Baldwins Gardens
London EC1N 7RJ

Tel: 020 7404 6609

www.pcaw.co.uk

ROYAL PHARMACEUTICAL SOCIETY

66-68 East Smithfield, London E1W 1AW

Tel: 0845 257 2570

www.rpharms.com

UNISON

UNISON Centre, 130 Euston Road
London NW1 2AY

Tel: 0845 355 0845

www.unison.org.uk

1 *www.parliament.uk/business/committees/committees-a-z/commons-select/health-committee/news/11-07-26-nmcreportpublished/*

2 *The healthcare regulators are: General Chiropractic Council; General Dental Council; General Medical Council; General Optical Council; General Osteopathic Council; Health Professions Council; Nursing and Midwifery Council; General Pharmaceutical Council and Pharmaceutical Society of Northern Ireland. The social care regulators are the Care Council in Wales; General Social Care Council in England; Northern Ireland Social Care Council and the Scottish Social Services Council.*

3 *These include, within the hospital setting, the Care Quality Commission in England, the Health Inspectorate Wales, Healthcare Improvement Scotland and the General Pharmaceutical Council if the concern is about registered pharmacy premises.*

APPENDIX 7: GPhC GUIDANCE ON MAINTAINING CLEAR SEXUAL BOUNDARIES

February 2012

ABOUT THIS GUIDANCE

This guidance should be read alongside the standards of conduct, ethics and performance which all pharmacists and pharmacy technicians must apply to their practice. This document gives guidance on standard 3.9 of the standards of conduct, ethics and performance, which says:

You must maintain proper professional boundaries in your relationships with patients and others you come into contact with during the course of your professional practice and take special care when dealing with vulnerable people.

STATUS OF THIS GUIDANCE

This document gives guidance to pharmacy professionals on the importance of maintaining clear sexual boundaries, and explains the responsibilities pharmacy professionals have. We have based this guidance on the Professional Standards Authority (PSA) document '**Clear sexual boundaries between healthcare professionals and patients: responsibilities of healthcare professionals**'[1].

You must make sure that all staff members you are responsible for are aware of this guidance and appropriately trained in all areas that are relevant to their duties.

If you are not sure about what you should do in a specific situation, you should always ask for advice from your employer, professional indemnity insurance provider, professional body or other pharmacy organisation, or get independent legal advice.

[1]*PSA: Clear sexual boundaries between healthcare professionals and patients: responsibilities of healthcare professionals: **www.professionalstandards.org.uk**.*

1. WHY IT'S IMPORTANT TO MAINTAIN CLEAR SEXUAL BOUNDARIES

1.1 When healthcare professionals cross professional boundaries the result for patients can be serious and can cause lasting harm. If you cross these boundaries it can damage public trust and confidence in the pharmacy profession and other healthcare professions.

1.2 Patients must be able to trust that you will act in their best interests. If you are sexually, or inappropriately, involved with a patient, your professional judgement can be affected. This involvement may affect the decisions that you make about their healthcare.

2. POWER IMBALANCE

2.1 The PSA (Professional Standards Authority) document explains that 'an imbalance of power is often a feature in the healthcare professional/patient relationship, although this may not be explicit'.

2.2 Patients are often vulnerable when they need healthcare. In the relationship between a patient and a healthcare professional, there is often a power imbalance. This may be because the patient shares personal information with you or because you have information and resources (such as medicines) that the patient needs. The patient may not be familiar with the situation they are in, or know what is appropriate professional behaviour. Therefore they may not be able to properly judge that the patient/professional relationship, or what happens to them, is appropriate. It is your responsibility to be aware of the imbalance of power and to maintain clear boundaries at all times.

2.3 You should always be clear with the patient about the reason for an examination or why you want them to come into the consultation room. Give them all the information they need and the opportunity to ask questions, and get their consent before going ahead.

3. SEXUALISED BEHAVIOUR AND BREACHES OF SEXUAL BOUNDARIES

3.1 The PSA document defines sexualised behaviour as 'acts, words or behaviour designed to arouse or gratify sexual impulses or desires'.

3.2 A breach of sexual boundaries is not limited to criminal acts, such as rape or sexual assault. For example, carrying out an unnecessary physical examination or asking for details of sexual orientation when it is not necessary or relevant, would both be a breach.

4. AVOIDING BREACHES OF SEXUAL BOUNDARIES

4.1 There are a number of behaviours that may be signs of showing sexualised behaviour towards patients or carers. These include:

- When the healthcare professional reveals intimate personal details about themselves to a patient during a consultation
- When the reason behind the following actions is sexual:
  - Giving or accepting social invitations (dates and meetings)
  - Visiting a patient's home without an appointment
  - Meeting patients outside of normal practice, for example arranging appointments for a time when no other staff are in the pharmacy
  - Asking questions unrelated to the patient's health.

4.2 If you find yourself in a situation where you are attracted to a patient, you must not act on these feelings. If you have concerns that this may affect your professional judgement, or if you are not sure whether you are abusing your professional position, you may find it helpful to discuss this with someone else. You might discuss this with an impartial colleague, a pharmacy organisation that represents you, a professional leadership body or your professional indemnity insurance provider.

4.3 If you cannot continue to care for the patient and be objective, you should find other care for the patient. You must make sure there is a proper handover to another pharmacy professional and that the patient does not feel that they are in the wrong as a result of your actions.

4.4 There may be situations when patients or their carers are attracted to you. If a patient shows sexualised behaviour towards you, you should think about whether you should discuss their feelings in a constructive way and try to re-establish a professional relationship. If this is not possible, you should transfer the patient's care to another pharmacy professional. You may find it helpful to discuss the matter with a colleague, a pharmacy organisation that represents you, a professional leadership body or your professional indemnity insurance provider.

5. CHAPERONES

5.1 A chaperone is a person (usually the same sex as the patient) who is present as a safeguard for the patient and the healthcare professional. They are also a witness to the patient's continuing consent for the procedure. Their role may vary depending on the needs of the patient, the pharmacy professional and the examination or procedure being carried out.

5.2 You should ask the patient whether they would like a chaperone to be with them in the consultation room, and for any examination that they might consider to be intimate. You should discuss the need for a chaperone with the patient and should not guess what their wishes are.

5.3 You should record any discussion that you have with patients about chaperones, including when the patient says that they do not want to have a chaperone present.

5.4 If no chaperone is available you should offer to delay and re-arrange the consultation or examination until one is available (unless a delay is not in the patient's best interests).

6. CULTURAL AND OTHER DIFFERENCES

6.1 Cultural differences can affect a patient's view of their personal boundaries and what is appropriate. You need to be sensitive to this, and always treat patients as individuals in a way that respects their views and maintains their dignity. For example, an individual may prefer to talk to or be examined by a pharmacy professional of the same gender, or have another person present.

7. PREVIOUS PATIENTS OR CARERS

7.1 The same principles apply to patients or carers that you have dealt with in the past and are not your patients any more. The previous professional relationship may also have involved an imbalance of power, and so would affect any personal relationship. If you think that this type of relationship may develop, you should consider the consequences or any harm this may cause to the patient and the impact on your professional standing. We advise you to consider the following:

- How long the professional relationship lasted and when it ended

- The nature of the previous professional relationship and whether it involved a significant imbalance of power

- Whether the former patient or carer was, or is, vulnerable

- Whether you are using the knowledge or influence that you gained through the professional relationship to develop or continue the personal relationship

- Whether you are already treating, or are likely to treat, any other members of the former patient's or carer's family.

7.2 It is your responsibility as a pharmacy professional to act appropriately and professionally, even if the relationship is agreed by everyone involved. You must consider all the issues above and, if necessary, get appropriate advice.

8. RAISING CONCERNS

8.1 You have a professional duty to raise concerns if you believe the actions of other individuals are putting patients at risk. This would include when you are concerned that clear sexual boundaries have not been maintained by other healthcare professionals. You must also take appropriate action if others report concerns to you.

8.2 See our document 'Guidance on raising concerns' for more information.

9. OTHER USEFUL SOURCES OF INFORMATION

- Clear sexual boundaries between healthcare professionals and patients: responsibilities of healthcare professionals, PSA: **www.professionalstandards.org.uk**

- Chaperone Framework, PSNC: **www.psnc.org.uk**

APPENDIX 8: GPhC GUIDANCE ON THE PROVISION OF PHARMACY SERVICES AFFECTED BY RELIGIOUS AND MORAL BELIEFS

September 2010

The General Pharmaceutical Council is the regulator for pharmacists, pharmacy technicians and registered pharmacy premises in England, Scotland and Wales. As part of our role, we set the standards which govern the practice of pharmacists and pharmacy technicians.

This document provides guidance on standard 3.4 of the standards of conduct, ethics and performance which states:

You must make sure that if your religious or moral beliefs prevent you from providing a service, you tell the relevant people or authorities and refer patients and the public to other providers.

This document gives guidance to pharmacy professionals on what they need to do if their religious or moral beliefs affect the provision of pharmacy services to patients and the public. Pharmacy professionals may also need to consider their contractual obligations, such as the NHS Terms of Service, if they are unable to provide a service.

This document also provides guidance to employers on what they need to do if they employ a pharmacy professional whose religious or moral beliefs may affect a service they provide.

NB: The GPhC has agreed that this provision will be reviewed during the first 12 months of operation.

1. GUIDANCE FOR PHARMACY PROFESSIONALS

Failure to provide specific pharmacy services will affect patients and the public, colleagues, employers and service commissioners. It is essential that relevant persons are informed and that patients and the public are directed to other service providers.

If your beliefs prevent you from providing a pharmacy service you should:

BEFORE ACCEPTING EMPLOYMENT

1.1 Think about where you are going to work and if the services you object to providing will be available and accessible in that vicinity. You need to remember that you must make patients your first concern.

1.2 Find out:

- If you will be working on your own or with other pharmacy professionals who will be able to provide the service

- Where you would direct patients requesting the service

- Whether the service you intend to direct patients to will be accessible and readily available to them at the time you will be on duty.

1.3 Tell employers, relevant authorities and the colleagues you will be working with about your beliefs. The persons or authorities who need to be informed may include:

- The superintendent pharmacist, pharmacy owner, pharmacist manager or other person responsible for employing pharmacists

- Locum agencies from whom you are seeking employment

- The primary care organisation or other body with whom you or the owner has a contract for services.

RESPONDING TO REQUESTS FOR A SERVICE

1.4 You are responsible for ensuring that the patient is properly informed about why the service they are requesting is not available. Be open and honest about your reasons for not providing a service as this will help patients understand and maintain trust and confidence in the profession.

1.5 Handle the situation sensitively. In some cases the initial request for a service will be made to another member of the pharmacy team so make sure that all staff are aware of your views and are trained to deal with the initial requests for services affected by your beliefs.

1.6 Respect the patient's right to confidentiality and take all reasonable steps to ensure appropriate levels of privacy for patient consultations even when you are unable to provide a service.

1.7 Patients should not be discouraged from seeking further information or advice.

Remember:

- If you do not supply emergency hormonal contraception (EHC) (either over the counter or against a prescription), women should be referred to an alternative appropriate source of supply available within the time limits for EHC to be effective

- If you do not supply routine hormonal contraception, women should be referred to an alternative appropriate source of supply available within the time period which will not compromise the woman's contraceptive cover

- If you refer a patient to a doctor's surgery or hospital you should think about whether the patient will be seen by a doctor or other appropriate practitioner within the timeframe required for treatment to be effective (i.e. consider factors such as the practice's opening hours and whether the patient will be able to get there)

- If you refer a patient to another pharmacy, check that there will be a pharmacist available there who can provide the service and that they have the relevant stock.

2. GUIDANCE FOR EMPLOYERS

Before you employ a pharmacy professional check whether they have any beliefs that prevent them from providing a particular pharmacy service. You must consider whether patients could be directed to alternative providers of the affected service in the vicinity. When you employ pharmacy professionals whose beliefs prevent them from providing a pharmacy service, you should:

2.1 Be satisfied that enough information has been given to the pharmacy professional about the services provided at the pharmacy in which they are going to work.

2.2 Have policies and procedures to guide staff in managing requests for services affected by moral and religious beliefs so that requests are handled appropriately and patients are able to access the services they require. Clear information on alternative services must be provided.

2.3 Ensure staff members are appropriately trained and provide them with the contact details and availability of local providers of the affected services.

APPENDIX 9: GPhC GUIDANCE FOR OWNERS AND SUPERINTENDENT PHARMACISTS WHO EMPLOY RESPONSIBLE PHARMACISTS

APPENDICES

September 2010

ABOUT THIS GUIDANCE

The General Pharmaceutical Council is the regulator for pharmacists, pharmacy technicians and registered pharmacy premises in England, Scotland and Wales. As part of our role, we set the standards which govern the practice of pharmacists and pharmacy technicians.

This document provides guidance on the standards for pharmacy owners and superintendent pharmacists of retail pharmacy businesses in relation to the responsible pharmacist regulations.

STATUS OF THIS GUIDANCE

This document gives guidance to owners and superintendent pharmacists on what they need to do when they employ a responsible pharmacist.

This guidance only relates to your responsibilities as a pharmacy owner or superintendent pharmacist in relation to the responsible pharmacist regulations and does not cover your other duties and obligations.

This document does not give legal advice and you must ensure that you comply with the relevant legislative requirements set out in:

■ The Medicines Act 1968

■ The Medicines (Pharmacies) (Responsible Pharmacist) Regulations 2008

■ Contractual obligations, such as the NHS Terms of Service.

I. APPOINTING AND SUPPORTING THE RESPONSIBLE PHARMACIST

In order to lawfully conduct a retail pharmacy business, a registered pharmacist must be in charge of the registered pharmacy as the responsible pharmacist.

YOU MUST:

1.1 Ensure that arrangements are in place to appoint a responsible pharmacist to be in charge of each registered pharmacy for which you are the owner or superintendent pharmacist. A pharmacist can only be the responsible pharmacist in charge of one registered pharmacy at any one time.

1.2 Ensure that arrangements are in place so that only a registered pharmacist who is competent and able to secure the safe and effective running of the registered pharmacy is appointed as the responsible pharmacist.

1.3 Ensure that the overarching operational framework for the registered pharmacy is established.

1.4 Support the responsible pharmacist in complying with their legal and professional duty to secure the safe and effective running of the registered pharmacy.

1.5 Enable the responsible pharmacist to comply with their legal and professional duty to secure the safe and effective running of the registered pharmacy. This includes allowing the responsible pharmacist to exercise their professional judgement.

2. THE PHARMACY RECORD

The pharmacy record is an important legal document. It shows who the responsible pharmacist is on any given date and at any time. This audit trail is particularly important in the event of any incident or error as it shows who was accountable. The pharmacy record may be kept in writing, electronically or in both forms. An entry in the pharmacy record may be made remotely as long as the record complies with all the relevant professional and legal requirements.

YOU MUST:

2.1   Ensure that the responsible pharmacist maintains the pharmacy record.

2.2   Ensure that the pharmacy record is kept for at least five years. For electronic records this is five years from the day the record was created. For written records this is five years from the last day to which the record relates.

2.3   Ensure that appropriate measures are in place to ensure that:

- The record is backed up

- The record is available at the premises for inspection

- Any alterations to the record identify when, and by whom, the alteration was made

if the pharmacy record is maintained electronically.

2.4   Ensure that the pharmacy record is available at the registered pharmacy for inspection by the responsible pharmacist, the pharmacy staff and our Inspectorate.

APPENDIX 10: GPhC GUIDANCE FOR RESPONSIBLE PHARMACISTS

September 2010

ABOUT THIS GUIDANCE

The General Pharmaceutical Council is the regulator for pharmacists, pharmacy technicians and registered pharmacy premises in England, Scotland and Wales. As part of our role, we set the standards which govern the practice of pharmacists and pharmacy technicians.

This document provides guidance on standard 7.7 of the standards of conduct, ethics and performance which states:

You must make sure that you keep to your legal and professional responsibilities and that your workload or working conditions do not present a risk to patient care or public safety.

STATUS OF THIS GUIDANCE

This document gives guidance to pharmacists on what they need to do if they are going to take on the role as the responsible pharmacist in charge of a registered pharmacy.

This document does not g ive legal advice and you must ensure that you comply with the relevant legislative requirements set out in:

- The Medicines Act 1968
- The Medicines (Pharmacies) (Responsible Pharmacist) Regulations 2008
- Any contractual obligations, such as the NHS Terms of Service.

I. SECURING THE SAFE AND EFFECTIVE RUNNING OF THE REGISTERED PHARMACY

In order to lawfully conduct a retail pharmacy business, a registered pharmacist must be in charge of the registered pharmacy as the responsible pharmacist.

The operational activities that may take place in the registered pharmacy when you are in charge of the pharmacy depend on the level of supervision provided and whether or not you are absent from the registered pharmacy. Examples of operational activities and the level of supervision required can be found in Appendix A.

YOU MUST:

1.1 Establish the scope of the role and responsibilities you will have as the responsible pharmacist and take all reasonable steps to clarify any ambiguities or uncertainties with the pharmacy owner, superintendent pharmacist or other delegated person.

1.2 Only take on the role of the responsible pharmacist if this is within your professional competence.

1.3 Only be the responsible pharmacist in charge of one registered pharmacy at any given time.

1.4 Secure the safe and effective running of the pharmacy business at the registered pharmacy in question before the pharmacy can undertake operational activities. Only after you are personally satisfied that you have secured the safe and effective running of the pharmacy can any operational activities begin to take place (see Appendix A).

2. DISPLAYING THE NOTICE

The notice is important as it allows patients and the public to identify the pharmacist who is responsible for the safe and effective running of the registered pharmacy. The details of the information that must be included on the notice can be found in Appendix B.

YOU MUST:

2.1 Conspicuously display a notice in the registered pharmacy.

3. THE PHARMACY RECORD

The pharmacy record is an important legal document. It shows who the responsible pharmacist is on any given date and at any time. This audit trail is particularly important in the event of any incident or error as it shows who was accountable.

The pharmacy record may be kept in writing, electronically or in both forms. An entry in the pharmacy record may be made remotely as long as the record complies with all the relevant professional and legal requirements.

The details that must be recorded in the pharmacy record are provided in Appendix C.

YOU MUST:

3.1 Ensure the pharmacy record is accurate and reflects who the responsible pharmacist is, and was, at any given date and time (including whether or not the responsible pharmacist is, or was, absent from the registered pharmacy).

3.2 Personally make the entries in the pharmacy record.

3.3 Ensure any amendments or alterations identify when, and by whom, the alteration was made, if the pharmacy record is maintained as a paper-based record.

3.4 Be satisfied that appropriate measures are in place to ensure that:

- The record is backed up
- The record is available at the registered pharmacy for inspection
- Any alterations to the record identify when, and by whom, the alteration was made

if the pharmacy record is maintained electronically.

3.5 Not become the responsible pharmacist or make an entry in the pharmacy record until you have secured the safe and effective running of the pharmacy business at the registered pharmacy in question.

3.6 Ensure that the pharmacy record is available at the registered pharmacy.

3.7 Ensure that the pharmacy record is available for inspection by the person who owns the pharmacy business, the superintendent pharmacist (in the case of a body corporate), the responsible pharmacist, the pharmacy staff and our Inspectorate.

4. PHARMACY PROCEDURES

The pharmacy procedures form part of the quality framework for the safe and effective running of the registered pharmacy. The pharmacy procedures may be maintained in writing, electronically or in both forms.

The matters that must be covered by the pharmacy procedures are provided in Appendix D.

YOU MUST:

4.1 Establish, if not already established, maintain and review pharmacy procedures.

4.2 Maintain adequate back-ups of the content of pharmacy procedures.

4.3 Ensure that the pharmacy procedures are available for inspection by the person who owns the pharmacy business, the superintendent pharmacist (in the case of a body corporate), the responsible pharmacist, the pharmacy staff and our Inspectorate.

4.4 Ensure that the pharmacy staff understand the pharmacy procedures that are in use.

4.5 Ensure that the pharmacy procedures:

- Are reviewed at least once every two years or following any incident or event that occurs which indicates that the pharmacy is not running safely and effectively
- Identify the responsible pharmacist who reviewed the procedures
- Identify which procedures are currently in place
- Identify which procedures were previously in place.

4.6 Make a temporary amendment to pharmacy procedures if the circumstances in the pharmacy change and in your professional opinion it is necessary to change the way in which the pharmacy normally operates.

4.7 Ensure there is an audit trail to identify:

- Which procedures are currently in place
- Which procedures were previously in place
- The responsible pharmacist who amended the procedure, and
- The date on which the amendment was made

if you make a temporary amendment to the pharmacy procedures.

5. ABSENCE

The responsible pharmacist may be absent for up to a maximum period of two hours during the pharmacy's business hours between midnight and midnight. If there is more than one responsible pharmacist in charge of the registered pharmacy during the pharmacy's business hours, the total period of absence for all the responsible pharmacists concerned must not exceed two hours.

Only certain operational activities (see Appendix A) may be undertaken in the pharmacy if the responsible pharmacist in charge of the registered pharmacy is absent.

IF YOU ARE ABSENT YOU MUST:

5.1 Remain contactable with the pharmacy staff where this is reasonably practical and be able to return with reasonable promptness, where in your opinion this is necessary to secure the safe and effective running of the pharmacy.

5.2 Arrange for another pharmacist to be available and contactable to provide advice to your pharmacy staff for any period of absence where it is not reasonably practicable to remain contactable and return with reasonable promptness.

APPENDIX A – Examples of operational activities and the level of supervision required

A1 Activities which require a responsible pharmacist to be in charge of the premises (they may be absent for up to two hours per day), and need to take place under the supervision of a pharmacist and the supervising pharmacist will need to be physically present at the premises. This is not an exhaustive list.

ACTIVITY	UNDERPINNING LEGISLATION	OTHER REGULATORY CONSIDERATIONS
PROFESSIONAL CHECK (CLINICAL AND LEGAL CHECK) OF A PRESCRIPTION	The professional check is not required under the Medicines Act 1968. The responsible pharmacist / superintendent responsibilities covered by Sections 70, 71, 72 and 72A of the Medicines Act 1968	The check is required under NHS pharmaceutical services legislation
SALE/SUPPLY OF PHARMACY MEDICINES	Sections 52, 70, 71, 72 and 72A of the Medicines Act 1968	'Supervision' in this context requires physical presence and a pharmacist being able to advise and intervene
SALE/SUPPLY OF PRESCRIPTION-ONLY MEDICINES (E.G. HANDING DISPENSED MEDICINES OVER TO A PATIENT, PATIENT REPRESENTATIVE OR A DELIVERY PERSON)	Sections 52, 58, 70, 71, 72 and 72A of the Medicines Act 1968	'Supervision' in this context requires physical presence and a pharmacist being able to advise and intervene
SUPPLY OF MEDICINES UNDER A PATIENT GROUP DIRECTION	Sections 52, 58, 70, 71, 72 and 72A of the Medicines Act 1968. Articles 12A-12E of the Prescription Only Medicines (Human Use) Order 1997	'Supervision' in this context requires physical presence and a pharmacist being able to advise and intervene
WHOLESALE OF MEDICINES	Section 10(7) of the Medicines Act 1968	'Supervision' in this context requires physical presence and a pharmacist being able to advise and intervene
EMERGENCY SUPPLY OF A MEDICINE(S) AT THE REQUEST OF A PATIENT OR HEALTHCARE PROFESSIONAL	Sections 52, 58, 70, 71, 72 and 72A of the Medicines Act 1968. Article 8 of the Prescription Only Medicines (Human Use) Order 1997	'Supervision' in this context requires physical presence and a pharmacist being able to advise and intervene

RPS note: the Medicines Act 1968 has been consolidated with the bulk of medicines legislation sitting within the Human Medicines Regulations 2012.

A2 Activities which require a responsible pharmacist to be in charge of the premises (they may be absent for up to two hours per day) and take place under the supervision of a pharmacist but who may not need to be physically present at the premises. This is not an exhaustive list.

ACTIVITY	UNDERPINNING LEGISLATION	OTHER REGULATORY CONSIDERATIONS
THE ASSEMBLY PROCESS (INCLUDING ASSEMBLY OF MONITORED DOSAGE SYSTEMS) ▪ Generating a dispensing label ▪ Taking medicines off the dispensary shelves ▪ Assembly of the item (e.g. counting tablets) ▪ Labelling of containers with the dispensing label ▪ Accuracy checking.	Section 10(1)(a) of the Medicines Act 1968	'Supervision' in this context may not require the physical presence of a pharmacist. The level of supervision required of the suitably trained staff who undertake this work will depend on what is regarded as good practice within the pharmacy profession (see the note in this Appendix below)

A3 Activities which require a responsible pharmacist to be in charge of the premises (they may be absent for up to two hours) but does not require the supervision of a pharmacist. This is not an exhaustive list.

ACTIVITY	UNDERPINNING LEGISLATION	OTHER REGULATORY CONSIDERATIONS
SALE OF GENERAL-SALE LIST MEDICINES	Sections 51, 70, 71, 72 and 72A of the Medicines Act 1968	Undertaken by suitable trained staff and operating within an agreed documented operating procedure

EXPLANATION OF 'ASSEMBLY'

The assembly of medicines against a prescription is controlled by Section 10 of the Medicines Act 1968.

In relating to a medicinal product 'assembly' is defined by the Medicines Act 1968 as:

enclosing the product (with or without other medicinal products of the same description) in a container which is labelled before the product is sold or supplied, or, where the product (with or without other medicinal products of the same description) is already enclosed in the container in which it is to be sold or supplied, labelling the container before the product is sold or supplied in it

Section 10 of the Medicines Act 1968 requires that the assembly process takes place under the 'supervision' of a pharmacist.

Supervision is not defined in the Act, and since the time the legislation was written the nature of assembly has changed in many instances. The introduction of patient packs has reduced the need to pack down or break bulk and the act of assembly often involves 'picking' the product rather than creating the final package or extemporaneously preparing medicines. The skills and competencies of staff undertaking dispensing activities have been developed and there is more emphasis of making full use of support staff releasing time for the pharmacist to provide a wider range of services. However, the legal definition remains the same.

The courts have considered the issue of the nature of 'supervision' required for the purposes of sale or supply of medicines and have concluded that, where supervision by a pharmacist is required, the actual transaction cannot take place without the physical presence of a pharmacist who is able to advise and intervene, even though s/he will not need to carry out the transaction themselves. However, the level of supervision required for assembly activities is less clear, and so for these activities, reference has to be made to more general case law of what 'supervision' means in the context of professional supervision.

The general position (derived from the Court of Appeal's judgement in Summers v Congreve Horner & Co [1992] 2 EGLR 152) is that supervision, in the context of professional supervision, means the degree of supervision required by what is regarded as good practice within the profession, having regard to the qualifications and experience of the person being supervised, but actual physical presence may not be necessary.

Applying that to the present context, it means that if the pharmacist responsible for supervising assembly of a medicinal product is absent, pharmacy support staff may continue to carry out activities which are considered to be 'assembling' activities for the purposes of the definition set out above, without breaching the legislation, provided it is recognised good practice within the pharmacy profession that they be allowed to do so. The Royal Pharmaceutical Society publishes good practice guidance, but it is important to emphasise that no single solution fits all circumstances. What may be good practice for one type of assembling activity may not be good practice for other types of assembling activities, and all such activities must be 'supervised' at an appropriate level.

It is also important to emphasise that this does not affect the position that the supply of assembled medicines against a prescription is prohibited unless the pharmacist is physically present in the registered pharmacy and in a position to advise and intervene. However, 'supervision' is not a 'one size fits all circumstances' legal concept, and the courts have recognised this.

APPENDIX B – The notice

The information that must be included on the notice is:

B1 Your name

B2 Your registration number

B3 That you are the responsible pharmacist in charge of that registered pharmacy premises

APPENDIX C – The pharmacy record

The details that must be recorded in the pharmacy record are:

C1 The responsible pharmacist's name

C2 The responsible pharmacist's registration number

C3 The date and time at which the responsible pharmacist became the responsible pharmacist

C4 The date and time at which the responsible pharmacist ceased to be the responsible pharmacist

C5 In relation to any absence of the responsible pharmacist from the registered pharmacy premises:

- The date of the absence
- The time at which the absence commenced; and
- The time at which the responsible pharmacist returned to the registered pharmacy premises.

APPENDIX D – Pharmacy procedures

The matters which must be covered by pharmacy procedures are:

D1 The arrangements to secure that medicinal products are:

- Ordered
- Stored
- Prepared
- Sold by retail
- Supplied in circumstances corresponding to retail sale
- Delivered outside the pharmacy
- Disposed of

in a safe and effective manner.

D2 The circumstances in which a member of pharmacy staff who is not a pharmacist may give advice about medicinal products

D3 The identification of members of pharmacy staff who are, in the view of the responsible pharmacist, competent to perform certain tasks relating to the pharmacy business

D4 The keeping of records about the arrangements mentioned in paragraph D1

D5 The arrangements which are to apply during the absence of the responsible pharmacist from the premises

D6 The steps to be taken when there is a change of responsible pharmacist at the premises

D7 The procedure which is to be followed if a complaint is made about the pharmacy business

D8 The procedure which is to be followed if an incident occurs which may indicate that the pharmacy business is not running in a safe and effective manner

D9 The manner in which changes to the pharmacy procedures are to be notified to pharmacy staff

APPENDIX 11: GPhC GUIDANCE ON RESPONDING TO COMPLAINTS AND CONCERNS

September 2010

The General Pharmaceutical Council is the regulator for pharmacists, pharmacy technicians and registered pharmacy premises in England, Scotland and Wales.

This document provides guidance on dealing with complaints and concerns raised by patients, the public and other healthcare professionals.

We are providing this guidance to assist pharmacy professionals on how to best meet the responsibilities that a pharmacy owner or pharmacy professional has in relation to handling and managing complaints and concerns.

As dispensing errors are frequently the basis for complaints, we will also provide guidance on:

- How to minimise the risk of a dispensing error occurring
- What to do in the event of a dispensing error
- How to review dispensing errors.

This Guidance Note has been published by the Standards Advisory Team. If you have questions about its content, please contact us on 020 3365 3460 or via email at standards@pharmacyregulation.org.

This Guidance Note will next be reviewed in October 2011.

INTRODUCTION

The standards of conduct, ethics and performance must be followed by pharmacists and registered pharmacy technicians. Principle 1 of these standards is to 'make patients your first concern'. A requirement under this principle is to 'organise regular reviews, audits and risk assessments to protect patient and public safety and to improve your professional service'.

The standards also require you to have standard operating procedures (SOPs) in place which must be followed at all times.

The standards for pharmacy owners and superintendent pharmacists of retail pharmacy businesses require

pharmacy owners and superintendent pharmacists to ensure the safe and effective running of the pharmacy. To allow this there must be appropriate policies, procedures and records in place that are maintained and reviewed regularly. There must also be an appropriate mechanism in place to respond to and investigate all complaints and concerns raised.

The standards referred to above can be found at **www.pharmacyregulation.org.**

WHY COMPLAINTS ARISE

There are numerous reasons for why a complaint or concern may arise. The majority of complaints or concerns are due to:

- Human error
- System failure, for example when a pharmacy doesn't have adequate SOPs in place
- How a complaint or concern is handled in the pharmacy.

The way in which a complaint or concern is handled in the pharmacy can determine whether or not it is then referred to an independent body such as the General Pharmaceutical Council (GPhC) or the primary care organisation (PCO).

HOW TO DEAL WITH A COMPLAINT OR CONCERN THAT HAS BEEN RAISED

When something goes wrong or someone reports a concern to you, you should make sure you deal with it appropriately.

There should be an effective complaints procedure where you work and you must follow it at all times.

You should make a record of the complaint, concern or incident and the action taken. You should review your records and findings and audit them regularly.

DISPENSING ERRORS

The investigating committee considered 732 cases between April 2009 and March 2010. Approximately 32% of these cases concerned dispensing errors. The Disciplinary Committee considered 396 cases during the same period of which 15% concerned dispensing errors.

HOW TO MINIMISE THE RISK OF MAKING A DISPENSING ERROR

DISPENSARY LAYOUT:

- The dispensary should be organised to keep distractions to a minimum
- The atmosphere of the dispensary should encourage good concentration
- Alert staff to the dangers of stock being placed in the wrong location. Dispensary stock should only be put away by a competent member of staff
- Keep a segregated area of the dispensary workbench for the dispensing process
- Segregate prescriptions on the workbench to avoid patients receiving someone else's medicines. You may use baskets/trays if appropriate.

DISPENSING PROCESS:

- Produce dispensing labels before any product is selected from the shelf
- Do not select stock using dispensing labels or patient medication records (PMR). Refer to the prescription when selecting stock for dispensing
- Dispense items from the prescription and not the generated label
- You should have systems in place to identify who was involved in the dispensing and checking process of each prescription item (e.g. dispensed by/checked by boxes)
- Two people should be involved in the dispensing process where this is possible. A second competent person should carry out an accuracy check and ideally should not have been involved in the assembly process
- If you are a pharmacist working alone, once you have assembled the medicines, try to create a short mental break between the assembly and final check to avoid carrying over any recollection of preconceived errors from the assembly process

- All accuracy checks should be made against the original prescription re-reading the prescription first
- Dispense balances of medication owed by reference only to the original prescription or a good quality copy. Do not rely solely on the information in the PMR or an owing note or label. This will prevent you making the same error that may have previously been made by another pharmacist.

The National Patient Safety Agency (NPSA) **(www.npsa.nhs.uk)** has published a document entitled 'A guide to the design of dispensed medicines', which looks at the key aspects of labelling and presentation of a dispensed medicine.

Another publication, entitled 'A guide to the design of dispensing environments', provides guidance on how the design of a dispensary can improve patient safety. Whilst the physical design of the dispensary can inevitably improve the working environment and therefore patient safety other things should also be considered. For example, the workflow and how the dispensary area is utilised can improve the efficiency and improve safety.

WHAT TO DO IN THE EVENT OF A DISPENSING ERROR

Pharmacists should carry out a root cause analysis in the event of a patient safety incident. This is a retrospective technique for looking for the underlying causes of a patient safety incident, behind the immediate and obvious cause. For example, one individual's human error might be the immediate cause, but several factors could have contributed to the error such as fatigue, an inadequate checking system or poor standard operating procedures.

The NPSA is promoting root cause analysis and is encouraging organisations to identify the circumstances in which it should be used. This should take into account the severity of the incident and the scope for learning from it. Further information on root cause analysis can be found on the NPSA website at **www.npsa.nhs.uk**.

You may wish to consider all the points below when dealing with an error or handling a complaint. In addition, locum pharmacists may also wish to keep their own records in case they are contacted later.

When the patient first comes in or indicates that there has been an error:

■ **ESTABLISH IF THE PATIENT HAS TAKEN ANY OF THE INCORRECT MEDICINE**

If the patient has taken any of the incorrect medicine, establish whether the patient has been harmed. If they have been harmed, provide the complainant and the patient's GP with the advice they need immediately. Contact the local drug information centre, if appropriate, for advice on the possible effects on the patient (giving details of concurrent medication). Where no harm appears to have been caused, the GP should still be informed.

■ **ASK TO INSPECT THE INCORRECT MEDICINE**

Make it clear that you do not wish to retain the medication, and that inspecting the medicine can give valuable clues about what went wrong. If the patient does not want to hand the medicine over to you, suggest that they retain it until they can hand it over to an appropriate representative of the GPhC or their local PCO. Incorrect medicines should not routinely be posted to these organisations.

If the patient does hand over and leave the incorrect medication with you retain it and keep it segregated from stock and other medicines to be supplied to patients.

Never dispose of any medicine unless the patient has given consent. Before doing so it should be retained carefully, for a reasonable period, in case of further developments.

■ **APOLOGISE**

In the case of a dispensing error, an apology should not be confused with an admission of liability.

■ **NEVER TRY TO MINIMISE THE SERIOUSNESS OF AN ERROR**

A balance must be struck that reassures the patient, if no harm is likely, but without suggesting that the error is insignificant.

■ **MAKE A SUPPLY OF THE CORRECT MEDICINE ORDERED ON THE PRESCRIPTION, IF APPROPRIATE**

You can lawfully make a supply of the correct medicine as this was authorised on the original prescription, even in the case of a Controlled Drug. Where the patient has not taken any of the incorrect medication it is your professional judgement about whether the patient's GP needs to be informed.

■ **ESTABLISH THEIR EXPECTATIONS**

It is important to establish what the complainant would like you to do about their complaint.

■ **PROVIDE DETAILS OF HOW TO COMPLAIN TO AN 'OFFICIAL BODY' IF REQUESTED**

Supply the complainant with the name and address of the Fitness to Practise Department of the GPhC if the complainant feels that the only way forward is to complain to an 'official body'. Explain that a Professional Standards Inspector from the GPhC may visit the pharmacy to undertake a review. You may also provide the details of the PCO so that the matter can be dealt with under the NHS complaints procedure.

■ **TRY AND ESTABLISH WHAT HAPPENED AND WHAT WENT WRONG**

You may need to make your own inquiries into any possible causes of the alleged error for preventative purposes unless it is clear from the facts known to you, how the error is likely to have occurred. You may need to speak to the person who presented or collected the prescription about the prevailing conditions in the pharmacy. Contact the complainant and inform them of your findings.

■ **FOLLOW COMPANY PROCEDURES / SOPS FOR REPORTING ERRORS OR COMPLAINTS**

Where you are an employee pharmacist, you should follow the procedures laid down by your employer/ Superintendent for who you should notify in the event of a dispensing error. If you are working within a company, you may have to report any errors to your line manager and/or a Superintendent office. You must follow company procedures for such reporting and may wish to consult the superintendent pharmacist and other line managers for advice.

■ **RECORD, REVIEW AND LEARN FROM ERRORS MADE**

See section on reviewing errors.

■ **NOTIFY THE PHARMACIST WHO WAS ON DUTY AT THE TIME, IF IT WAS NOT YOU**

You may use the Responsible Pharmacist record to ascertain who was on duty at the time.

■ **INFORM YOUR PROFESSIONAL INDEMNITY INSURANCE PROVIDER**

In all cases of dispensing errors, the over-riding responsibility is for the health and well-being of the patient. Whilst keeping this in mind, you should inform your professional indemnity insurers as soon as possible, in case a claim is later made against you.

REVIEWING ERRORS

Make a written record of your findings when you carry out your review to establish what went wrong. You can record your findings using the mnemonic 'CHAPS' to cover the various areas of the supply. CHAPS covers the following points:

C CONDITIONS IN THE PHARMACY AT THE TIME

This can be established from the:

- Complainant
- Records – records would help to identify the name of the responsible pharmacist and whether they had been working without a break
- Computer – computer records may help to identify the number of prescriptions dispensed that day and the exact time the prescription was dispensed.

Interestingly, most errors do not occur during busy periods of dispensing.

You may wish to review the layout of the dispensary and the availability of bench space. You may use baskets or similar to hold dispensed items before checking and handing to the patient with counselling. It has been reported that pharmacists who use this type of system help prevent medicines being crossed from one patient to another, and also to keep the bench space tidy.

H HEALTH OF THE PHARMACIST AND OTHER MEMBERS OF THE TEAM

Was the pharmacist or other person(s) involved in the dispensing process ill at the time?

A ASSISTANCE

Was the pharmacist working alone or was s/he assisted? Identify the person who assisted. Make a judgement about the qualifications and competence of the assistant.

P PRESCRIPTION SHOULD BE RECOVERED FROM THE FILE OR GET A COPY OF IT FROM THE RELEVANT PRESCRIPTION PRICING AUTHORITY

- Was the error caused by the legibility of the prescription?
- Was the prescription hand written or computer generated?
- Check endorsements for what was supplied.

S SYSTEMS USED FOR DISPENSING AND CHECKING MUST BE REVIEWED

Depending upon whether the pharmacist was working alone or with someone assisting, this covers every part of the dispensing process. The type of error may direct your attention to one area of dispensing practice.

Usually errors fall into categories:

- Misreading the prescription
- Incorrect picking of the medicines
- Transposing the label or labelling the medicine incorrectly
- Giving the wrong prescription to the wrong patient (for example, where the error involves placing the medicine in the wrong bag or where the patient's address is not checked properly when handing out the dispensed medicine)
- Selection of the wrong strength (or wrong preparation) from the PMRs when using the repeats facility, then checking the stock against the label, not the original prescription
- Incorrect compounding
- Supplying contaminated or out-of-date stock
- Dispensing against an incorrectly written owing slip, rather than the prescription.

Whatever weaknesses there are in the system, the final accuracy check must overcome them. It is most important to review these critically.

The mnemonic 'HELP' can be used when making the final check on the dispensed medicine, to ensure that all the necessary checks have been made. HELP stands for the following:

H 'HOW MUCH' HAS BEEN DISPENSED

Open all unsealed cartons and sealed cartons, if appropriate, to check that the contents are correct and match the quantity requested on the prescription. Check that the correct patient information leaflet has been included.

E 'EXPIRY DATE' CHECK

Ensure this is sufficient to cover the treatment period.

L 'LABEL' CHECK

Check the patient's name, product name, form, strength and dose are the same as on the prescription. Check that the correct and appropriate warning(s) are included on the label.

P 'PRODUCT' CHECK

Check that the correct medication and strength which has been requested on the prescription has been supplied.

Handing out of dispensed medicines must be carried out by trained staff. To avoid handing medicines to the wrong person, prescription receipts may provide useful safeguards, although even these are not foolproof. The person collecting the dispensed medicine should be asked for the address or date of birth of the patient, which should be checked against the prescription.

When reviewing dispensing errors which have resulted in a serious patient safety incident, the NPSA incident decision tree helps to identify why individuals acted in a certain way, and this may be a very useful tool for pharmacists, managers and organisations to consider using. Information on the incident decision tree can be found at **www.npsa.nhs.uk.**

APPENDIX 12: GPhC GUIDANCE FOR REGISTERED PHARMACIES PREPARING UNLICENSED MEDICINES

May 2014

ABOUT THIS GUIDANCE

This guidance should be followed if an unlicensed medicine is prepared in a registered pharmacy. The preparation of an unlicensed medicine (for example unlicensed methadone, or menthol in aqueous cream) in a pharmacy is often called 'extemporaneous preparation'.

The guidance should be read alongside the **standards for registered pharmacies**[1]. These aim to create and maintain the right environment, both organisational and physical, for the safe and effective practice of pharmacy.

By following this guidance the pharmacy will:

- Demonstrate that it meets our standards, and
- Provide assurances that the health, safety and wellbeing of patients and the public are safeguarded.

Responsibility for making sure this guidance is followed lies with the pharmacy owner. If the registered pharmacy is owned by a 'body corporate' (for example a company or an NHS organisation) the superintendent pharmacist also has responsibility. Those responsible for the overall safe running of the pharmacy need to take into account the nature of the pharmacy and the range of services already provided and, most importantly, the needs of patients and members of the public.

As well as meeting our standards, the pharmacy owner and superintendent pharmacist must make sure they keep to all legal requirements, including medicines legislation, and health and safety, data protection and equalities legislation.

Pharmacy owners and superintendent pharmacists should make sure that all staff, including non-pharmacists, involved in preparing unlicensed medicines are familiar with this guidance.

Individual pharmacy professionals are key to ensuring the safe preparation and supply of unlicensed medicines. Pharmacists and pharmacy technicians involved in preparing unlicensed medicines have a responsibility[2]

to provide medicines safely to patients, maintain the quality of their practice, keep their knowledge and skills up to date, and work within their professional competence.

We expect this guidance to be followed. However, we also recognise that there can be a number of ways to meet our standards and achieve the same outcomes for patients – that is, to provide safe treatment, care and services. If you do not follow this guidance, you should be able to show how your alternative ways of working safeguard patients, identify and manage any risks, and meet our standards.

In this document, when we use the term 'you' this means:

- A pharmacist who owns a pharmacy as a sole trader, and
- A pharmacist who owns a pharmacy as a partner in a partnership, and
- A pharmacist who is the appointed superintendent pharmacist for a body corporate, and
- The body corporate itself.

THE SCOPE OF THIS GUIDANCE

This guidance applies only to the process of preparing[3] an unlicensed medicine by (or under the supervision of) a pharmacist in a registered pharmacy in Great Britain, under the exemptions and circumstances described in the law[4]. It applies whether this happens rarely, occasionally or is part of the core business of the registered pharmacy.

---

1 Standards for registered pharmacies

2 Standards of conduct, ethics and performance

3 This guidance does not apply to unlicensed medicines that registered pharmacies have not prepared themselves, but have obtained from elsewhere such as (MS) licensed manufacturers, importers or distributors

4 Section 10 of the Medicines Act 1968 and Regulation 4 of the Human Medicines Regulations 2012

This guidance applies to all the following:

- The one-off preparation of an unlicensed medicine in accordance with a prescription for an individual patient

- The preparation of a stock[5] of unlicensed medicines, (in anticipation of a prescription), which will later be supplied from the pharmacy, by or under the supervision of a pharmacist, against a prescription for an individual patient

- The preparation of methadone for supply in accordance with a prescription (either for immediate supply in accordance with the prescription, or initially as stock[5] to be supplied from the pharmacy, by or under the supervision of a pharmacist, against a prescription at a later time)

- The preparation of an unlicensed medicine based upon the pharmacist's judgement[6]

- The preparation of an unlicensed medicine by, or under the supervision of, a pharmacist based on the specification of the patient.

If the activity is not covered by the exemptions set out in the law, you will need a Manufacturer's Specials (MS) licence from the Medicines and Healthcare products Regulatory Agency (MHRA).

If the medicines are being prepared for animal use, the exemptions that allow this, and the parts of the law that apply, are found in the Veterinary Medicines Regulations 2013. The body that regulates animal medicines and issues authorisations to manufacturers of special veterinary medicinal products is the Veterinary Medicines Directorate (VMD).

Throughout this document we use the terms 'preparing' and 'preparation' which refer to making a medicine from ingredients or starting materials. These terms are not intended to include the process of simply diluting or dissolving a product in a vehicle designed for that purpose as part of its marketing authorisation – for example, adding a set amount of water to reconstitute an antibiotic powder.

5 Preparation for stock at a pharmacy is acceptable as long as it is subsequently supplied by retail from that pharmacy or another pharmacy which is part of the same legal entity

6 An unlicensed medicine that is prepared with the intention of selling it over the counter (one that is not a prescription-only medicine) is often called a 'Chemist's Nostrum'

7 Medicines Act 1968 and the Human Medicines Regulations 2012

8 www.mhra.gov.uk

9 www.gmc-uk.org

INTRODUCTION

The law[7] sets out the restrictions on how human medicines are licensed, manufactured, advertised, administered, sold and supplied.

Most of the medicines supplied from registered pharmacies are licensed medicines. Licensed medicines are those that have a valid Marketing Authorisation (MA) in the UK, and which are covered by an approval process overseen by the MHRA.

The manufacturers who make these medicines are also regulated and licensed by the MHRA for compliance with EU Good Manufacturing Practice (GMP) standards and the strict conditions of their licence. You can find more information about the approval and inspection of manufacturers on the MHRA's website[8].

These arrangements mean that licensed manufacturers are making medicines to a regulated standard that is consistent throughout the industry. It also means that when medicines are used in line with their licence, they are:

- Assured to a certain level of efficacy, quality and safety, and

- Only available if they are effective.

Overall this means that the public, and patients, can have a high degree of confidence that appropriately prescribed licensed medicines are effective and meet the clinical needs of patients.

As a rule, the law requires that only authorised (licensed) medicines should be made available and supplied ('placed on the market'). There are exemptions in the law which allow unlicensed medicines to be prescribed and supplied to individual patients.

In general, when a prescriber issues a prescription they will prescribe a medicine that is licensed and indicated for the condition to be treated. European and UK law sets out the circumstances under which prescribers can prescribe an unlicensed medicine for supply to a patient. You can find more information on the prescribing of an unlicensed medicine by reading the General Medical Council's (GMC's) *Good practice in prescribing and managing medicines and devices* on their website[9].

Under the law, unlicensed medicines ('special products') must be manufactured by the holders of MS ('specials') licences who are regulated by the MHRA and who follow GMP standards and the conditions of their licences.

In general, the law also requires the medicine itself be licensed[10]. However, the law[11] allows a pharmacist to prepare and supply medicines in a registered pharmacy without the need for the product to be licensed. A pharmacist should have acquired the necessary knowledge and skill during their initial education and training leading to registration.

A patient has every right to expect that when an unlicensed medicine is prepared by, or under the supervision of, a pharmacist in a registered pharmacy, it is of an equivalent quality to any licensed medicine they will receive (such as those produced by a regulated and licensed manufacturer). As certain high-profile past cases[12] have shown, preparing an unlicensed medicine in a pharmacy is an activity that can pose a significant risk to patients and have potentially serious consequences when risks and processes are not managed properly.

When a patient is supplied with an unlicensed medicine, it is important that the unlicensed medicine is safe and appropriate. Pharmacists making supplies must also consider their individual professional standards and their responsibilities to the patient. There is also a general legal duty that all medicines supplied to patients are of the nature and quality requested or prescribed.

The law also allows a pharmacist in a registered pharmacy to prepare medicines for animal use in line with a prescription, prescribed under the cascade[13], from a veterinary practitioner.

The authorised specials manufacturers of veterinary medicines are inspected by the VMD for their compliance with the principles of GMP. If they manufacture human medicines they would also be regulated by the MHRA.

If you choose to prepare unlicensed medicines in your pharmacy under the exemptions in the law, you should follow the guidance set out in this document.

10 *Regulations 17 and 46 of the Human Medicines Regulations 2012*

11 *Section 10 of the Medicines Act 1968 and Regulation 4 of the Human Medicines Regulations 2012*

12 *Peppermint water case*

13 *Veterinary Medicines Regulations 2013*

The owner and the superintendent pharmacist are responsible for making sure that there are systems in place to safeguard the health, safety and wellbeing of patients and the public who use their services. This guidance covers the areas we believe may present an increased risk when medicines are prepared in a registered pharmacy. It will help the owner, and superintendent pharmacist, to meet our standards for registered pharmacies.

GUIDANCE FOR REGISTERED PHARMACIES PREPARING UNLICENSED MEDICINES

The standards for registered pharmacies are grouped under five principles, and this guidance is set out under each of those five principles.

PRINCIPLE 1

The governance arrangements safeguard the health, safety and wellbeing of patients and the public. The following areas relate to this principle in the standards for registered pharmacies.

1.1 RISK ASSESSMENT

A risk assessment is a careful and thorough look at what, in your work, could cause harm to patients and what you need to do to prevent this. Risk assessments should be specific to the individual pharmacy, the staff working in it, and to each unlicensed medicine to be prepared.

You should consider the risks before deciding whether your pharmacy should prepare unlicensed medicines in general, or whether you might consider other options for supplying particular medicines.

You should carry out a risk assessment if an unlicensed medicine is prepared in your pharmacy, and carry out the necessary checks to satisfy yourself that any arrangements you have in place to manage the risks involved meet the requirements of principle 1. If your intention is that your pharmacy will prepare medicines, you will need to be able to produce evidence for the arrangements you have in place to manage the risks identified.

The risk assessment should be reviewed regularly (see section 1.2) and should also be reviewed when circumstances change (see section 1.3).

The risk assessment should state what the risks are, and may include finding out whether equivalent relevant licensed products exist and are available.

While this is not a full list of issues that need to be taken into account, the assessment should, if applicable, look at:

- A formula from a recognised source, for example from an official Pharmacopoeia
- A verification of the preparation method (eg the Pharmacopoeia method)
- A calculation verification
- The use of specialist equipment
- Consideration of contamination
- Hygiene measures
- Product-specific risks
- Assurances around ingredients and starting materials
- The suitability of premises
- Relevant staff skills
- Training and competence
- The circumstances that would trigger a new risk assessment.

1.2 REGULAR AUDIT

You should have robust systems in place so that you can demonstrate that your pharmacy:

- Continues to be a safe place in which to prepare unlicensed medicines for patients, and
- Can produce medicines which are safe, effective and of a suitable quality.

You should carry out a regular audit, at an interval that you can show to be appropriate, on the process of preparing unlicensed medicines. The audit should form part of the evidence which provides assurance and shows that the pharmacy continues to be safe and appropriate to carry out this activity.

While this is not a full list of issues that need to be taken into account, the audit should, if applicable, look at:

- The premises (including temperature, light and moisture controls and where applicable – for example in aseptic preparation – air quality and other environmental requirements)
- The equipment and facilities
- The preparation process and quality control
- The hygiene issues that might have an adverse impact on the product and therefore the patient (including avoiding cross-contamination and microbial contamination)
- Staff training and skills

- The records (including the method of preparation, traceability of ingredients used, labelling applied and how the records themselves are kept).

You should learn from any incidents, complaints or other forms of relevant information and use the learning to make appropriate changes.

1.3 REACTIVE REVIEW

A review should take place when any of the following happens:

- Changes in key staff (those who have specialist training, knowledge and experience and are involved in preparing medicines)
- The introduction of new staff
- A change in the equipment
- A change in the form, or source, of ingredients
- Any incidents
- The environment or facilities available are no longer fit for the task
- Concerns or feedback received
- A review of near misses and error logs indicates concerns about this activity.

This reactive review, which should be documented, should say when a new risk assessment is needed. It can form part of that new risk assessment, when one needs to be carried out.

1.4 RECALL PROCEDURES

It is important that if there is a problem with an unlicensed medicine that has been prepared in your pharmacy, you have the systems in place to contact members of the public and recall unlicensed medicines that have been made in your pharmacy.

These procedures should say who is responsible for taking action, and what action to take. They should also include details of the other bodies or authorities that need to be told about the medicines' recall.

Under the standards you must have arrangements in place that allow all staff to raise concerns when they suspect that medicines are not fit for purpose.

1.5 ACCOUNTABILITY – STAFF

It should be clear which pharmacist is accountable and responsible for the preparation of an unlicensed medicine.

It should also be clear which pharmacy technician and other staff are involved in preparing an unlicensed medicine.

1.6 RECORD KEEPING

You should keep detailed records of the preparation of the unlicensed medicine to safeguard patients. This is so that if there is a recall, or an incident affecting a patient's safety, the method of preparation can be clearly reconstructed.

You should keep records for as long as you consider, and can show, to be appropriate, taking into account any consumer protection laws which apply. If the medicine being prepared is for animal use there are specific requirements in the law for record keeping that also apply. Ask the pharmacy's professional indemnity insurance provider for advice about how long you should keep records for.

The records should include information on the following:

THE PROCESS	Description of the key preparation steps used
	Calculations: working shown and double checked (detailed)
	The name of the person who prepared the worksheet
	The date that the worksheet was prepared
	The name of the supervising pharmacist (and the name of the pharmacist signing off the final product as ready to be supplied to the patient, if different)
	The name of the pharmacy technician involved (if applicable)
THE FORMULA	The complete formula
	The source of the formula: Pharmacopoeia formula or other source
	Validation of the formula
THE INGREDIENTS (FOR EACH INGREDIENT OR STARTING MATERIAL USED)	The source: manufacturer, brand and the wholesaler or distributor
	Certificate of conformity[14] (if applicable)
	Certificate of analysis[15] (if applicable)
	Batch number
	Expiry date (if available)
	Quantity used and details of the person measuring, and person double-checking, quantities
	TSE guidance[16] should be followed (if applicable, that is, where an ingredient or product contact material is of animal origin)
	Description of the container and closure used (for example whether they were glass or plastic)

14 Certificate of conformity provides confirmation that the product supplied complies with a specified set of requirements or specifications, but does not contain any test results

15 Certificate of analysis provides a summary of testing results on samples of products or materials together with the evaluation for compliance to a stated specification

16 The TSE guidance is the MHRA guidance: 'Minimising the Risk of Transmission of Transmissible Spongiform Encephalopathies via Unlicensed Medicines for Human Use'. See the Other sources of information section at the end of this document for more information

THE PRODUCT	Date prepared
	A reference number or identification (batch number)
	Expiry date (give reasons or validation in support)
	Date supplied to the patient or customer

THE PATIENT OR CUSTOMER	The patient or customer's name
	The patient or customer's address
	The patient or customer's contact details (for example, phone number, email address)
	A sample of the label that has been put on the medicine
	The name of the person who produced the label

(ALSO, IF SUPPLIED AGAINST A PRESCRIPTION)	The patient's doctor (name, address and phone number)
	The patient's age (if it is on the prescription)
	Other prescription details (date and type)

INCIDENTS	Suspected adverse reactions reported
	Complaints and concerns

PRINCIPLE 2

Staff are empowered and competent to safeguard the health, safety and wellbeing of patients and the public.

The following areas relate to this principle in the standards for registered pharmacies.

2.1 TRAINED AND COMPETENT STAFF

Staff should complete recognised training courses before they can be involved in this activity. However, staff may also be involved in this activity if they are still doing such a training course, but their work in this area must be closely supervised until their training is complete.

To prepare an unlicensed medicine from ingredients, staff need expertise and skill over and above that needed to dispense a licensed medicine. Many pharmacists and pharmacy technicians should have acquired this knowledge and skill during their initial education and training leading to registration. If they do not have the necessary knowledge, skills or competence to safely carry out the task, you should consider how you ensure that they obtain (or if they have previously been trained in this area, refresh) the necessary specialist skills.

It is important that training is regularly repeated to make sure that all staff remain up to date and competent. This is particularly important when the activity is only carried out from time to time.

Staff working with potentially hazardous substances (such as cytotoxic products), or in areas that require more stringent precautions (such as aseptic preparation), should have done specific, recognised and relevant training.

2.2 TRAINING RECORDS

You should document and keep evidence of the training done for as long as you consider, and can show, to be appropriate. These records should be made available to the relevant authorities if they ask for them.

You should ask the pharmacy's professional indemnity insurance provider for advice on how long you should keep records for.

PRINCIPLE 3

The environment and condition of the premises from which pharmacy services are provided, and any associated premises, safeguard the health, safety and wellbeing of patients and the public.

You should assess the risks and consider whether your pharmacy premises are suited to, and capable of, providing this service. You should get specialist advice when you are considering preparing sterile (aseptic) or hazardous medicines (for example cytotoxics, hormones or immunosuppressants).

There are highly specialised requirements for the safe preparation of aseptic medicines, and there are potentially significant adverse consequences to patients if there is an error with, or contamination of, these medicines. You should get specialist advice from a body such as the MHRA or regional NHS Quality Assurance staff (some of which also operate on a consultancy basis and can provide services across Great Britain and to non-NHS organisations too).

See the *Other sources of information* section at the end of this document for more information on this subject.

The following areas relate to this principle in the standards for registered pharmacies.

3.1 MEASURES TO MINIMISE CONTAMINATION

There should be enough space, and segregation where required, to provide this service safely, and the environment of the premises should be suitable for the preparation of medicines.

Specific steps should be taken to make sure that the risk of cross-contamination and microbial contamination is eliminated or minimised within the pharmacy.

These factors should be considered as part of the initial risk assessment.

See the *Other sources of information* section at the end of this document for links to information provided by governmental infection control agencies.

3.2 HYGIENE CONTROL RECORDS

You should make records of the steps taken to make sure that the environment, conditions and equipment are clean enough for the preparation of medicines. These will form part of the evidence that the pharmacy is suitable for the preparation of unlicensed medicines.

You should keep the records for as long as you consider, and can show, to be appropriate. You should ask the pharmacy's professional indemnity insurance provider for advice on how long you should keep records for.

PRINCIPLE 4

The way in which pharmacy services are delivered safeguards the health, safety and wellbeing of patients and the public. This includes the management of medicines and medical devices.

The following areas relate to this principle in the standards for registered pharmacies.

4.1 INGREDIENTS

The ingredients and starting materials used in the preparation of the unlicensed medicine will affect the quality of the final product. Therefore you should make sure that any ingredients or starting materials your staff use are obtained from a reputable source: for example, a licensed manufacturer or distributor.

4.2 QUALITY ASSURANCE

Quality assurance, in this context, is the procedures, processes and arrangements in place that make sure a finished medicine is of the quality needed for its intended use.

To have a robust system of quality assurance that provides the necessary safeguards, you need to have a range of systems in place, such as those described in this guidance. These include:

- Using worksheets and official formulas
- Confirmation of quantities and identities of ingredients
- Staff whose training is suitable and up to date, and
- Appropriately maintained equipment.

You should have procedures in place which include a specific method, process, or system that is used consistently to assure yourself that the unlicensed medicine produced is of suitable quality to be supplied to the patient.

When more than a single one-off preparation is made, this quality assurance should be robust enough to safeguard all the patients who may be supplied from a single batch of medicines.

4.3 PATIENT INFORMATION

At the outset, you should make sure that there is a system in place so that the Responsible Pharmacist (or other staff competent to be delegated this task) tells the patient that the pharmacy will be preparing an unlicensed medicine.

They should explain to the patient what this means (including what this means in relation to the amount of information and evidence available about the medicine).

When a pharmacy supplies an unlicensed medicine there is no legal requirement to give a package leaflet, or similar detailed written information. Therefore the patient will rely on the information that your pharmacy staff give them. You should give appropriate advice and information (in writing if possible). This applies equally when there is limited, or no, direct contact with the patient when the medicine is supplied.

You should make sure that the pharmacy staff give the patient any important information they might need so that they can use the medicine safely. The information should include advice on the use of any dosing device that needs explanation to deliver the correct dose. You should also make sure that pharmacy staff consider what extra information they should give the patient about the medicine: for example, the expiry date or any special storage instructions.

If the medicine is prepared in line with a British Pharmacopoeia (BP) formula or a general monograph in the BP for the dosage form, there are particular labelling requirements for unlicensed medicines.

There are also specific labelling requirements when the prepared medicine is for animal use, which has been prescribed by a veterinary practitioner under the cascade.

PRINCIPLE 5

The equipment and facilities used in the provision of pharmacy services safeguard the health, safety and wellbeing of patients and the public.

The following areas relate to this principle in the standards for registered pharmacies.

5.1 SPECIALIST EQUIPMENT AND FACILITIES

You should make sure that the pharmacy has equipment and facilities which are specially designed for the intended purpose that staff will use them for. They should be of sufficiently high specification, and accuracy where applicable, to produce a high-quality, safe product.

Examples of specialist equipment include, but are not limited to, the following:

- Accurate measuring devices for weight (measuring scales)
- Accurate measuring devices for volume (for example, cylinders)
- Production and mixing equipment
- Cleaning equipment (including suitable detergent)
- Contamination-minimising clothing (for example, masks, gloves, aprons, coats, hats)
- Sterilising equipment (including suitable chemical agents, autoclaves and filtration equipment)
- Fume cupboards, isolators and laminar flow cabinets.

5.2 MAINTENANCE LOGS

You should keep maintenance logs, including validation and calibration records, for each type of specialist equipment for as long as you consider, and can show, to be appropriate. These logs will form part of the evidence that the pharmacy is suitable for the preparation of medicines.

You should ask the pharmacy's professional indemnity insurance provider for advice on how long you should keep records for.

OTHER SOURCES OF INFORMATION

- *Rules and Guidance for Pharmaceutical Manufacturers and Distributors 2014 'The Orange Guide'* (or any subsequent revision). You can find more information on the MHRA's website
- *Minimising the Risk of Transmissible Spongiform Encephalopathies via Unlicensed Medicinal Products for Human Use* contains information for if an ingredient, or product contact material, of animal origin is used in the preparation of an unlicensed medicine
- *Veterinary Medicines Guidance Note No 13 Guidance on the Use of Cascade* contains information on the extemporaneous preparation of medicines
- The following agencies are a source of information on infection control: Health Protection Scotland; Public Health England; Health Protection Agency (for Wales).

Other references that may be useful and of interest include:

- *Handbook of Extemporaneous Preparation,* Ed. Jackson and Lowey on behalf of the NHS Pharmaceutical Quality Assurance Committee, Pharmaceutical Press, 2010
- *Quality Assurance of Aseptic Preparation Services Edition 4*, Ed. A.M. Beaney on behalf of the NHS Pharmaceutical Quality Assurance Committee, Pharmaceutical Press, 2006
- *PICIS Guide to Good Practices for the Preparation of Medicinal Products in Healthcare Establishments PE 010-3 2008*
- *Resolution CM/ResAP(2011)1.* The European Directorate for the Quality of Medicines and Healthcare has passed a resolution on quality and safety assurance requirements for medicinal products prepared in pharmacies for the special needs of patients.

MEDICINES, ETHICS AND PRACTICE

APPENDIX 13: GPhC GUIDANCE FOR REGISTERED PHARMACIES PROVIDING PHARMACY SERVICES AT A DISTANCE, INCLUDING ON THE INTERNET

April 2015

ABOUT THIS GUIDANCE

This guidance explains what you should consider before deciding whether any parts of your pharmacy service can be provided safely and effectively 'at a distance' (including on the internet), rather than in the 'traditional' way.

A 'traditional' pharmacy service is one where all parts of the pharmacy service, including the sale and supply of medicines, takes place in the same registered pharmacy. For example, the patient brings their prescription to the registered pharmacy, pharmacy staff dispense it and advise the patient in the same pharmacy.

Different ways of providing pharmacy services are becoming more common. We recognise that because of changes in society and advances in technology, pharmacy services will continue to adapt and change. However the pharmacy service is delivered, the legal principles and regulatory standards aimed at guaranteeing safe outcomes for patients and people who use pharmacy services must still be met. The sale and supply of Pharmacy (P) medicines and Prescription Only Medicines (POMs) must only happen at or from a registered pharmacy under the supervision of a pharmacist, even when the sale or supply is made on the internet.

To meet the needs of patients and people who use pharmacy services, some parts of the pharmacy service may not take place at the pharmacy itself. The authorisation to supply a P medicine or the clinical check of a prescription may take place off site. Examples of this would be at a clinic or care home, although the supply of medicines would still have to be from a registered pharmacy and supervised by a pharmacist.

We want this guidance to be useful for pharmacies wanting to innovate and introduce new ways of working. We also want it to support appropriate access to medicines and pharmaceutical care, which complies with the law and meets our standards.

You should read this guidance alongside the **standards for registered pharmacies**[1].

Following this guidance will help your pharmacy to:

- Meet our standards, and
- Provide assurances that the health, safety and wellbeing of patients and people who use pharmacy services are safeguarded.

The pharmacy owner is responsible for making sure this guidance is followed. If the registered pharmacy is owned by a 'body corporate' (for example a company or an NHS organisation) the superintendent pharmacist also has that responsibility. Those responsible for the overall safe running of the pharmacy must take into account the nature of the pharmacy, the range of services provided and, most importantly, the needs of patients and people who use pharmacy services.

As well as meeting our standards, the pharmacy owner and superintendent pharmacist must make sure they keep to all the laws that apply to pharmacies.
This includes the law on supplying and advertising medicines[2], new consumer information for online sales[3], and data protection[4].

---

1 www.pharmacyregulation.org/standards/standards-registered-pharmacies

2 www.gov.uk/advertise-your-medicines
https://www.gov.uk/government/publications/blue-guide-advertising-and-promoting-medicines

3 www.gov.uk/government/policies/providing-better-information-and-protection-for-consumers

4 www.ico.org.uk/for_organisations/sector_guides/health

Pharmacy owners and superintendent pharmacists should make sure that all staff involved in providing pharmacy services at a distance – including on the internet – are familiar with this guidance. All staff have a responsibility to provide medicines safely to patients and to only do work they are competent to do.

We expect this guidance to be followed. However, we also recognise there are a number of ways to meet our standards and achieve the same outcomes for patients and people who use pharmacy services – that is, to provide safe treatment, care and services. If you do not follow this guidance you must be able to show how your own ways of working:

- Safeguard patients and users of pharmacy services
- Identify and manage any risks, and
- Meet our standards.

In this document, when we use the term 'staff' this includes:

- Employees (registrants and non-registrants)
- Agency and contract workers, and
- Any third party who helps the pharmacy provide any part of the pharmacy service, and deals with patients and people who use pharmacy services on behalf of the pharmacy owner.

In this document, when we use the term 'you' this means:

- A pharmacist who owns a pharmacy as a sole trader, and
- A pharmacist who owns a pharmacy as a partner in a partnership, and
- A non-pharmacist who owns a pharmacy as a partner in a partnership in Scotland, and
- A pharmacist who is the appointed superintendent pharmacist for a body corporate, and the body corporate itself.

We will review this guidance from time to time, to make sure it stays relevant when there are changes in government policy or the law, or when new ways of working develop.

5 www.systems.hscic.gov.uk/eps

6 A collection and delivery service is defined in Regulation 248 of the Human Medicines Regulations 2012.

THE SCOPE OF THIS GUIDANCE

This guidance covers pharmacy services that are not 'traditional' ones. In a 'traditional' pharmacy all parts of the service are provided at the same registered pharmacy, including:

- Displaying medicines for sale
- Receiving prescriptions for dispensing
- Assessing whether Pharmacy (P) medicines and General Sale List (GSL) medicines, and prescriptions, are clinically appropriate
- Advising patients and people who use pharmacy services and counselling them on how to take their medicines
- Taking payments, prescription charges or notifications of exemption from patients
- Selecting medicines for supply
- Assembling, preparing and labelling medicines against prescriptions
- Handing over medicines to patients or their carers and representatives.

So this guidance applies to pharmacy services when any of the activities above are carried out at different registered pharmacies or places. It also applies in all cases when a member of staff or a third party providing any part of the pharmacy service, and the patient or person who uses the pharmacy service, are not both in the same registered pharmacy together.

Examples of the pharmacy services covered by this guidance include:

- A pharmacy service where prescriptions are not handed in by patients but collected by pharmacy staff, or received by post or electronically – such as in the electronic prescription service (EPS)[5]
- A delivery service from the registered pharmacy to patients in their own home or in a care home or nursing home
- A collection and delivery service[6]
- A 'click and collect' service
- A mail order service from a registered pharmacy
- An internet pharmacy service, including ones linked to an online prescribing service whether or not the prescribing service is owned and operated by you, or by a third party business

- A 'hub and spoke'[7] pharmacy service, where medicines are prepared, assembled, dispensed and labelled for individual patients against prescriptions at a central 'hub' registered pharmacy.

This is not a full list. You must consider how you will follow this guidance and meet our standards for registered pharmacies if you intend to provide any part of your pharmacy service at a distance, including on the internet. You need to make sure you identify and manage risks, and supply medicines and services safely to patients and people who use pharmacy services.

INTRODUCTION

The law[8] says that pharmacy (P) medicines and prescription-only medicines (POMs) can only be sold or supplied, or offered for sale or supply, from a registered pharmacy. And this must be done by, or under the supervision of, a pharmacist.

The law[9] also says that medicines can only be prepared, assembled, labelled and supplied for individual patients against prescriptions at a registered pharmacy under the supervision of a pharmacist.

This same law applies whether you provide pharmacy services in a 'traditional' way, at a distance or on the internet.

Even if you offer a delivery service, the handover to the delivery agent of a P or POM medicine must take place at a registered pharmacy under the supervision of a pharmacist.

If you sell or supply medicines to patients in other countries you must keep to any other laws that apply. This may include making sure the medicine you supply has the marketing authorisation needed for it in that country[10].

If you sell or supply medicines for animal use, the parts of the law that apply, and the exemptions that allow this, are covered elsewhere[11]. The Veterinary Medicines

Directorate (VMD)[12] licenses and approves animal medicines and issues guidance on supplying medicines for animals.

The NHS Regulations in England[13] include a number of specific situations that allow distance-selling pharmacies to open and operate. In Scotland and Wales the regulations are not the same. However, they do not prevent pharmacies that are already open from providing pharmacy services at a distance or on the internet.

GUIDANCE FOR REGISTERED PHARMACIES PROVIDING PHARMACY SERVICES AT A DISTANCE, INCLUDING ON THE INTERNET

The standards for registered pharmacies are grouped under five principles, and this guidance is set out under each of the five principles.

PRINCIPLE 1

The governance arrangements safeguard the health, safety and wellbeing of patients and the public.

1.1 RISK ASSESSMENT

There are different risks with providing any pharmacy service at a distance, including on the internet. Before you start providing the service, you should gather evidence that you have identified and managed the risks, and checked that the arrangements you have in place meet the requirements of principle 1. This will show you can provide the service safely and effectively.

A risk assessment will help you identify and manage risks. It is a careful and thorough look at what in your work could cause harm to patients and people who use pharmacy services, and what you need to do to keep the risk as low as possible. You may want to make sure that risks are reduced 'as low as reasonably practicable'[14], managing the risk against what you have to do to reduce it further.

7 The dispensed medicines are supplied by the 'hub' to 'spokes' or delivered direct to patients in their homes or to care homes. The 'spokes' may be other registered pharmacies; or non-registered premises, where patients drop off their prescriptions and from where they collect their dispensed medicines.

8 Regulation 220 of the Human Medicines Regulations 2012. Supplies made by hospitals, and made by doctors or dentists to their patients, are exempt from this.

9 Section 10 Medicines Act 1968. There are exemptions when these activities take place under the supervision of a pharmacist in a hospital, a care home or a health centre.

10 Regulation 28 of the Human Medicines (Amendment) Regulations 2013

11 Veterinary Medicines Regulations 2013

12 www.gov.uk/government/organisations/veterinary-medicines-directorate

13 The National Health Service (Pharmaceutical and Local Pharmaceutical Services) Regulations 2013

14 www.hse.gov.uk

Your risk assessment should say what risks you have identified, and include the different options you have for setting up your pharmacy service. Your staff should know the outcome of any risk assessment and contribute to it appropriately. If you keep a risk register, you are responsible for keeping it up to date and recording any actions you have taken.

Risk assessments may be corporate wide but still need to take into account the circumstances of each individual pharmacy, including the staff working in it, and each individual part of the pharmacy service you intend to provide. It should cover the whole service.

If parts of your pharmacy service are the responsibility of several different pharmacies and staff, you should consider how the systems you use to provide your pharmacy service work together – including IT systems for exchanging information between different locations. You should also consider how you monitor the accuracy of these systems and manage any potential failures.

Areas of risk you should think about include:

- How staff tell patients and the public about the pharmacy services they will receive, and how they get their consent

- How staff communicate between different locations

- Medicines supply, including counselling and delivery (see principle 4)

- Your business's capacity to provide the proposed services, and

- Business continuity plans, including website and data security.

Not all risks can be foreseen and dealt with in advance. Some may only appear with time, as a result of:

- Patient, user of pharmacy service or staff behaviour

- Different technologies operating together, or

- An increase in the number, or scale, of services.

You should therefore review your risk assessment regularly (see section 1.2), and when circumstances change – for example, when you make significant business or operational changes (see section 1.3).

1.2 REGULAR AUDIT

You should carry out a regular audit, at an interval that you can show to be appropriate, for your pharmacy services. You should also be able to show how your staff are involved in the audit. Regular audits may be corporate wide, but still need to be relevant to the circumstances of each individual pharmacy.

The audit should be part of the evidence which gives assurance and shows that your pharmacy continues to provide safe pharmacy services to patients and people who use those services. You should take action to sort out any issues you identify, and this may lead to your carrying out a 'reactive' review (see section 1.3).

This is not a full list of issues, but you should consider the following as part of your regular audit:

- Staffing levels and the training and skills within the team

- Suitability of communication methods with patients, and between staff and other healthcare providers, including between hubs and spokes and with collection and delivery points

- Systems and processes for receiving prescriptions, including EPS

- Records of decisions to make or refuse a sale

- Systems and processes for secure delivery to patients

- Any information about your pharmacy services on your website

- How you keep to your information security policy, Payment Card Industry Data Security Standard (PCI DSS) and data protection law

- Feedback from patients and people who use pharmacy services

- Concerns or complaints received, and

- Activities of third parties, agents or contractors.

You should consider whether your information security practices need to be audited by independent experts, depending on the type of service you provide.

1.3 REACTIVE REVIEW

You should carry out a review if a regular audit identifies a problem, or when any of the following happens:

- A change in the law affecting any part of your pharmacy service
- A significant change in any part of the pharmacy service you provide, for example an increase in the number of patients you provide services to, or an increase in the range of services you intend to provide
- A data security breach
- A change in the technology you use
- Concerns or negative feedback are received from patients or people who use pharmacy services
- A review of near misses and error logs causes a concern about an activity.

You should record this reactive review and say clearly when a new risk assessment needs to be carried out.

1.4 ACCOUNTABILITY – STAFF

When parts of a pharmacy service take place at different locations (such as in a 'hub and spoke' or 'click and collect' service) you must be clear about which pharmacist is accountable and responsible for each part of the service, and which pharmacy technician and other staff are involved.

When medicines are not given to the patient in the registered pharmacy but are delivered by a member of staff or an agent to the patient's home or workplace, there may be more risk of medicines being lost or delivered to the wrong person. You must make sure there are clear lines of accountability and responsibility in these circumstances.

If you contract out any part of your pharmacy service to a third party you are still responsible for providing it safely and effectively. You must carry out 'due diligence' in selecting any contractors.

1.5 RECORD KEEPING

You should decide, as part of your risk assessment, what records you keep depending on the nature of the pharmacy services you provide.

When a patient has direct face-to-face contact with pharmacy staff in a pharmacy no records of the sale of P medicines are usually made. And when a product is unsafe or unsuitable and no supply is made, staff tell the patient, but no records are usually kept.

When there is no face-to-face contact, you should consider what information you and your staff record and keep to show that the pharmacy service you provide is safe. This may include the key points on which you made the decision to sell or not to sell a particular medicine. The records you keep are important evidence for the judgements you and your staff make, and can be a powerful tool for service improvement and quality management.

Although medicines law says how long you should keep certain records, you should keep other records for as long as you consider, and can show, to be appropriate.

The records should include:

- Information on risk assessments, audits and reactive reviews
- Details of the staff accountable and responsible for providing each part of your pharmacy service
- The information and advice you give patients and people who use pharmacy services on using medicines safely
- Consent to use a particular delivery method, and the date of dispatch of the medicine
- Information on complaints or concerns from patients or people who use pharmacy services and what you have done to deal with these; and
- IT records (see principle 5).

PRINCIPLE 2

Staff are empowered and competent to safeguard the health, safety and wellbeing of patients and the public.

2.1 TRAINED AND COMPETENT STAFF

You are responsible for creating a culture of patient-centred professionalism within your pharmacies. This should support pharmacists and pharmacy technicians in behaving and practising as professionals. You must make sure that all staff are properly trained and competent to provide medicines and other professional pharmacy services safely. This is vital to the safety and wellbeing of patients and the public.

You must be able to show you have considered the specific training staff will need to provide any part of your pharmacy service. You and your staff must do any relevant training needed before being involved in providing any pharmacy services at a distance, including on the internet. Staff may be involved in these services while they are doing this training, but their work in this area must be closely supervised until their training is finished.

You should consider extra training in the following areas:

- Information security management – how patient data is protected, and cyber security
- Communication skills[15] to support staff in managing effective non-face-to-face communications with patients and prescribers, and
- Using specialised equipment and new technology.

You should document and keep evidence of the training done for as long as you consider, and can show, to be appropriate.

PRINCIPLE 3

The environment and condition of the premises from which pharmacy services are provided, and any associated premises, safeguard the health, safety and wellbeing of patients and the public.

3.1 YOUR PREMISES

You must make sure your pharmacy and the premises you use for any part of your pharmacy services meet the standards for registered pharmacies.

If you provide pharmacy services at a distance or on the internet, your registered pharmacy must be fit for purpose to reflect the scale of the work you do. If you automate certain activities, there must be enough space to use automated dispensing systems safely. You should make sure that you have suitable areas in your registered pharmacy to send medicines to patients safely.

3.2 YOUR WEBSITE

If you sell and supply P medicines on the internet, you must make sure that these are only displayed for sale on a website that is associated with a registered pharmacy. This could be under a service level agreement or some other arrangement. The public may be able to access the site directly or through a third-party site.

People who use pharmacy services should be able to select a P medicine for purchase only on a website associated with a registered pharmacy.

You should consider the design and layout of your website and make sure that it works effectively and looks professional.

Your website must be secure and follow information security management guidelines and the law on data protection. This is particularly important when you ask

patients for personal details. You must make sure that your website has secure facilities for collecting, using and storing patient details[16] and a secure link for processing card payments.[17]

All information must be clear, accurate and updated regularly, and it must not be misleading in any way. Your site may include information about medicines, health advice and links to other information sources such as relevant healthcare services and other regulators. Your site must not mislead pharmacy service users about the identity or location of the pharmacies involved in providing your pharmacy services.

Links from your pharmacy website to an online prescribing service or another registered pharmacy website must be clearly shown as such. Some pharmacy businesses and online prescribing services are owned by the same company and operate together using the same website. If you allow a link to another business (either hosted on your website or reached by an external link) you are responsible for making sure the business is legitimate. And, if relevant, it must be registered with the appropriate regulator such as the Care Quality Commission, Healthcare Improvement Scotland or the Health Inspectorate Wales.

You should display prominently on your website:

- The GPhC pharmacy registration number
- Your name as the owner of the registered pharmacy
- The name of the superintendent pharmacist, if there is one
- The name and address of the registered pharmacy that supplies the medicines
- Details of the registered pharmacy where medicines are prepared, assembled, dispensed and labelled for individual patients against prescriptions (if any of these happen at a different pharmacy from that supplying the medicines)

---

15 Support for professionals or employers wanting to develop communications skills of staff are available from a range of organisations referenced at the end of this guidance

16 See www.ico.org.uk/for_organisations/sector_guides/health

17 For example a secure link that complies with the Payment Card Industry Data Security Standard (PCI DSS)

- Information about how to check the registration status of the pharmacy and the superintendent pharmacist (if there is one)
- The email address and phone number of the pharmacy
- Details of how patients and users of pharmacy services can give feedback and raise concerns.

Later this year the MHRA will launch the compulsory EU internet logo[18]. When this is available you must apply to the MHRA for this logo and display it on every page of your website if you sell any GSL or P medicines, or supply POM medicines, on the internet. (The EU internet logo will also be displayed on the websites of non-pharmacy retailers of GSL medicines). You will need to meet all the conditions set out in the law[19] before the MHRA will give you the EU internet logo for display.

You may also apply to use the voluntary GPhC internet logo[20] on your website, which links directly to the GPhC register entry for your pharmacy. You can only display it on your own website. You must not allow it to be used by a third party, prescribing or other website.

PRINCIPLE 4

The way in which pharmacy services, including the management of medicines and medical devices, are delivered safeguards the health, safety and wellbeing of patients and the public.

4.1 TRANSPARENCY AND PATIENT CHOICE

Patients have the right to make decisions about their care and medicines, and the services they want to receive, including being able to choose where they want their medicines supplied from. Pharmacy professionals must give the patient the information they need so they can make an informed decision about their medicines and the pharmacy services they use.

Your pharmacy service can be associated with a medical or non-medical prescribing service. The prescribing service may be:

- One where you order and collect prescriptions on behalf of patients from the doctor's surgery, or
- One where you receive prescriptions by post or electronically, or
- An online service that patients can access on your pharmacy website or by a link from your pharmacy website.

In all cases, you and your staff must make sure patients consent to any pharmacy service you provide using these prescribing services.

You must be able to show that your arrangements with medical or non-medical prescribers are transparent, and do not:

- Cause conflicts of interest
- Restrict a patient's choice of pharmacy, or
- Unduly influence or mislead patients deliberately or by mistake.

If parts of your pharmacy services are provided at different locations you must explain clearly to patients and people who use pharmacy services where each part of the service is based. You must avoid any information that could mislead the patient or user of the pharmacy service about the identity or location of the pharmacy.

4.2 MANAGING MEDICINES SAFELY

Selling and supplying medicines at a distance, including on the internet, brings different risks than those of a 'traditional' pharmacy service. You should consider these as part of your initial risk assessment. (See also principle 1).

You should be able to show the steps you have taken to minimise the risks you identify. This should include how you:

- Decide which medicines are appropriate for supplying at a distance, including on the internet
- Make sure your pharmacy staff can:
  - Check that the patient is who they claim to be, and
  - Get all the information they need from patients to check that the supply is safe and appropriate, taking into account for example their age, gender, other medicines and other relevant issues
- Make sure patients can ask questions about their medicines
- Make sure patients know who to contact if they have any questions or want to discuss something with the pharmacy staff, and
- Identify requests for medicines that are inappropriate, too large or too frequent.

18 www.gov.uk/government/organisations/medicines-and-healthcare-products-regulatory-agency
19 Regulation 28 of the Human Medicines (Amendment) Regulations 2013
20 www.pharmacyregulation.org/registration/internet-pharmacy

4.3 SUPPLYING MEDICINES SAFELY

You should make sure the medicines are delivered safely to the correct person when they need them. You should consider how to do this as part of the initial risk assessment.

You should be able to show the steps you have taken to manage the risks you identify. This should include how you:

- Assess the suitability and timescale of the method of supply, dispatch, and delivery[21] (for example, for refrigerated medicines and controlled drugs)

- Assess the suitability of packaging (for example, packaging that is tamper proof or temperature controlled)

- Check the terms, conditions and restrictions of the carrier

- Check the laws covering the export or import of medicines if the intended recipient is outside the UK

- Train your staff, and

- Monitor third-party providers.

4.4 PATIENT INFORMATION

When pharmacy staff do not see the patient face to face you should consider how staff can communicate any important information to patients clearly and effectively.

You must also tell patients about services that take place at different locations, and you must make sure you have their consent for this form of service.

You must give clear information to patients and people who use pharmacy services on how they can contact your pharmacy staff if they have any problems or need more advice. This should also include advice on when they should go back to their GP or local pharmacist.

PRINCIPLE 5

The equipment and facilities used in the provision of pharmacy services safeguard the health, safety and wellbeing of patients and the public.

5.1 SPECIALIST EQUIPMENT AND FACILITIES

You should make sure that your pharmacy service has equipment and facilities which are specifically designed for the intended purpose, and your equipment is:

- Of high specification, accuracy and security, and

- Calibrated, maintained and serviced regularly in line with the manufacturer's specifications, and you keep maintenance logs for as long as you consider, and can show, to be appropriate.

Examples of specialist equipment include:

- Automated dispensing systems and labelling equipment

- Mobile devices used for remote access.

Your software for providing services at a distance, including on the internet, should be robust enough to handle the volume of work.

You must make sure your IT equipment meets the latest security specifications. You must also make sure the security of data is protected when it is in transit, by either wired or wireless networks, inside your business and outside it. You must also control access to records and how you store, keep and remove records.

---

21 Royal Pharmaceutical Society www.rpharms.com Delivery and posting of medicines to patients - Medicines, Ethics and Practice – The professional guide for pharmacists Edition 38 July 2014.

OTHER SOURCES
OF INFORMATION

CENTRE FOR POSTGRADUATE PHARMACY EDUCATION (CPPE)

Confidence in consultation skills
www.cppe.ac.uk/learning/Details.
asp?TemplateID=Consult-W-
02&Format=W&ID=115&EventID=-

COMMUNITY PHARMACY SCOTLAND

www.communitypharmacyscotland.org.uk

COMMUNITY PHARMACY WALES

www.cpwales.org.uk/Home.aspx

DEPARTMENT FOR BUSINESS, INNOVATION & SKILLS

www.getsafeonline.org/shopping-banking/buying-
medicines-online1/
www.cyberstreetwise.com/#!/protect-business/what-
you-need-to-know

EUROPEAN ALLIANCE FOR ACCESS TO SAFE MEDICINES (ASOP EU)

www.asop.eu/

HEALTH AND SOCIAL CARE INFORMATION CENTRE

www.systems.hscic.gov.uk/eps

MEDICINES AND HEALTHCARE PRODUCTS REGULATORY AGENCY

Falsified medicines directive: Sales of medicines at a distance to the public
www.gov.uk/government/organisations/medicines-and-
healthcare-products-regulatory-agency
www.ec.europa.eu/health/human-use/eu-logo/index_
en.htm

Risks of buying medicines over the internet
www.nidirect.gov.uk/risks-of-buying-medicines-over-
the-internet

NATIONAL PHARMACY ASSOCIATION (NPA)

www.npa.co.uk

NHS ENGLAND

www.england.nhs.uk/

PHARMACEUTICAL SERVICES NEGOTIATING COMMITTEE

www.psnc.org.uk/

Distance selling pharmacies
www.psnc.org.uk/contract-it/market-entry-regulations/
distance-selling-pharmacies/

Electronic prescription service
www.psnc.org.uk/dispensing-supply/eps/

ROYAL PHARMACEUTICAL SOCIETY

www.rpharms.com

VETERINARY MEDICINES DIRECTORATE

Internet retailers of veterinary medicines
www.vmd.defra.gov.uk/pharm/internetretailers.aspx

INDEX

INDEX

INDEX

MEDICINES, ETHICS AND PRACTICE